METAPHYSICAL HEALING

These lessons are the practical experience of Metaphysics applied to disease in all its aspects to restore Health on all planes, Physical, Astral, Mental, Soul and Spirit. They show how to master disease and gain and retain what the world is seeking, Equilibrium and Health

By

DR. A. S. RALEIGH

Volume I

A Course of Private Lessons given
to his personal pupils

THE HERMETIC PUBLISHING COMPANY

3006 Lake Park Ave.   Chicago, Ill., U. S. A.

Kessinger Publishing's Rare Reprints
Thousands of Scarce and Hard-to-Find Books!

We kindly invite you to view our extensive catalog list at:
http://www.kessinger.net

CONTENTS

LESSON ON

HEALTH AND DISEASE

Disease is from dis-ease, that is, a lack of harmony, or discord. Health is the reverse, namely Harmony. Harmony of what? — and discord of what? Of vibration of the system. Remember that the gross physical body is permeated by energies of a much more subtle form. These energies are in a continuous state of vibration. Never for one moment are they still, never do they become motionless, but it is ever a process of continuous motion, ever moving in accordance with the diverse rates of vibration. As the rate of vibration is, so will be the character of their influence. They are vibrating on the different octaves; the Mental Body, the Astral Body and the Etheric Double are each and all of them in this continuous state of vibration.

Motion is going on perpetually. This motion is either in accordance with harmony or else it is discordant. If it be discordant it will manifest itself in a disordered condition of the system; be it chronic or acute, it must at all times be a physical disturbance proportionate to the discord which has taken place in the vibrating energy of the system. This may be in the Astral Body, the Mental Body or the Etheric Double.

In every case Health is the result of harmony of the vibrating force; disease, the effect of discord. Not only is this true, but there are specific diseases which are the effects of specific kinds of discord, that is to say, specific degrees of discord in the manifesting vibrating force, but also a particular kind of discord, discordant in the sense that there are certain notes of inharmony manifesting themselves there. A certain type of discord must necessarily express itself in and through a given disease. The changing of this form of discord into some other form will consequently eventuate in a change of one type of disease into another. As the type of discord is, so will be the type of disease.

By either thinking in discord or feeling in discord, or also by

7

living in such a way physically that the Etheric Double vibrates in a discordant manner, we will establish this discordant state, which, descending to the Gross Body, establishes discord in the cells and thus will produce this state of inharmony, this state of disease, as we term it. Fevers, chills, rheumatism, neuralgia, malaria, in fact, everything, in a word every disease that flesh is heir to is but an expression of a definite form of discord.

It may occur to you to ask, "Well, isn't it a fact that the influence of our physical environment will produce disease?" Undoubtedly it will, because the physical environment will produce a state of discord. The vibration of the atmosphere may be inharmonious, there may be putrifying substances about which will produce discordant vibrations in the air, which will poison the food you eat, the water you drink, so that these, in turn, are discordant in their vibration. If this be true you will naturally take on this discordant influence and your principles will be made to move in the discordant manner that is prompted by the discordant influence around you. In this way you take on that condition, you develop that phase of discord and, in the course of time, it descends until the physical body is made to respond and you contact the disease. If you can maintain your harmony, however, in that environment in spite of the discord that is all around you, you will discover that you can maintain perfect health notwithstanding the diseases that are going on about you.

When you contact contagious diseases it is not due to the action of germs; it is due to a discordant auric force which sets up a corresponding discord in your own aura and this, descending, throws your system out of gear. The one who is able to preserve perfect harmony of vibration in his own aura, may go into the worst pest hole on earth with perfect impunity.

Poisons produce disease by reason of their ability to breed discordant conditions, but if one is so permeated with the spirit of harmony that nothing can disturb it, that no discordant element can ruffle this state of harmony the least bit in the world, he will find he can drink poison with impunity.

In the treatment of disease, it is, therefore, only necessary to establish a state of harmony instead of discord. If you can accomplish this result you will be able to cure any disease in the world. It is because of this fact that New Thought, Christian Science, the Science of Being — all those metaphysical cults, are so wonderfully successful. Analyze them and you will discover that their methods are mainly directed to the end of establishing a state of harmony, throughout the system. They work against any discordant element, and work to the end of harmonizing everything, and thus by producing this harmony of vibration, you will find they are establishing the state of health. Health is being continually suggested by this operation, by this activity, by the method which is adopted, and the result is, health and harmony are induced.

To bring out of this discord a state of harmony is, therefore, the cure for all the diseases to which flesh is heir and nothing else will cure them. This is the problem. The method which is adopted must work unto the accomplishment of that end. Methods are of value only as they lead unto the realization of this state of harmony. Any method which will accomplish this result is effective. A method which does not, should never be resorted to.

It should be borne in mind that if we know just what the rate of discord is, we may bring about the state of harmony much more easily than if we do not understand it. If we do not understand it we may try to bring it into harmony with a certain rate of vibration which is really much more antagonistic to it than some other. We must know the general character of the vibratory activities of the body and bring all the discordant states into harmony with them. We must also recognize the antipathies which exist between the human organism, particularly the organism of our patient, and certain influences, and thus avoid all such antipathies, acting through the sympathies rather.

To accomplish this work requires the skill of a Master and no one else should ever, at any time, attempt the healing of the body.

In the treatment of disease everything which will harmonize with the condition of the patient and bring about this state of harmony, must be resorted to. A careful study of the colors, of the character of perfumes, if the person wears them, all the arrangements about the house – everything must be conducive to HARMONY and must also harmonize with the condition of the patient. Nothing discordant should be permitted, because it will simply aggravate the disease.

It should also be borne in mind that the people with whom we associate exercise a great influence upon our being. They are likely to either harmonize with us or become antagonistic. Their auras may be out of harmony with our own. If so, it will have the tendency to establish a state of discord within our own being. Thus many people are made sick because of the company they keep, because of their families. As a matter of fact, one should never try to live with disagreeable people if he has any regard for his health. More people are made sick because their families, their friends are not agreeable, not congenial, than are ever made sick because of malaria germs, or anything of the kind. Do not have disagreeable people around if you would maintain a state of health, because they will necessarily disturb your emotional states and antagonize the entire being. The result will be a state of discord which must express itself in a corresponding disease. In order to cure a patient under such conditions it is necessary that he should be removed from those conditions which have given rise to that state of discord.

Also, it must be borne in mind that if a person within himself live a life of antagonism, a life of bitterness, of hatred, — maintain a discordant condition within his own being, then he is sinning against the Law of Harmony, the Law of Peace. The result is he is establishing that state of discord which must express itself in corresponding diseases, and so sickness is really the punishment for sin; it is the consequence which a life of discord brings, and sickness can never be permanently cured except by the permanent removal of the causes, namely, the state of Discord. Harmony must be produced within the very being before he can be brought into a state of permanent health.

Also remember what we call disease, those eruptions, so to speak, manifesting in the physical body, those types which are ordinarily termed disease, are merely the symptoms of the real evil which lies within. The real disease, remember, is a state of discord within the Aura — that is the enemy with which we have to contend. This expresses itself in a discordant state of the cellular structure of the body. The diverse organs, the tissues, even become disturbed and this disturbance arising, produces certain effects — usually because of the accumulation of effete matter in the system; because there is something there which is not proper from a physical standpoint, they manifest themselves in the ordinary way. But be that as it may, remember that the physical troubles which we try to cure are the effects of those discordant states in the vibration of the Aura, that being the REAL CAUSE, the physical disturbances that we call Disease being merely the outward expression, the effect, the excrescence, so to speak, of this inward state of discord, consequently the curing of the symptoms while the discord remains, will, in every instance, be found to produce no lasting benefit, but to simply "salve" the matter over. The elimination of the discord by the establishment of harmony, is the only permanent and rational cure of disease. It is in this sense that the dictum of New Thought is true, namely, that all physical troubles are the effects of mental troubles, and a diseased mind is the cause of a diseased body, therefore, cure the mind and you will cure the body.

If we understand that a disturbed, discordant Aura is the cause of all the influences detrimental to health, manifesting in the Gross Body, consequently that all physical troubles are the effects of Auric Disturbances, Auric Discord, we will then have the key to the situation. So the only radical method of treating disease is by establishing Harmony within the Aura, harmony of vibration throughout the finer principles of man's constitution. When you have accomplished this, you have accomplished a cure for all diseases.

Therefore, remember that Health is the inevitable result of an harmonious state of vibration throughout the finer principles. A discordant state of that vibration, where there is any antagonism, where one rate of vibration is contending with another, where there is independence in the vibration, half a dozen, or a dozen, each acting independently of the others, where there is the least disharmony, the least discordant influence, it must express itself in a disturbed state of the body which we call disease.

Also each specific type of discord represents itself in a corresponding disturbed condition. In other words, it is establishing a corresponding type of disease, a type corresponding to the type of discord which gives expression to it. Also this discord may be brought back into a state of harmony. Whenever it is, the disease disappears and becomes a state of health.

Lastly, Disease can be cured only by replacing Discord by Harmony, and when this is accomplished, it will be cured in every case, without fail, as disease cannot exist in a body nourished by an Aura vibrating in a state of Perfect Harmony. Any attempt to cure disease without recognizing it as being the effect of discord within the finer principles, any attempt, in a word, to cure by regarding disease as being a physical condition and not the effect of the higher conditions, must result in mere patchwork, which will, perhaps, remove one symptom, but allow the manifestation of discord through some other symptoms.

Health is HARMONY: — Disease is DISCORD. The problem of Therapeutics is the problem of replacing Discord by Harmony.

LESSON ON

ASTRAL CHEMISTRY

One of the most important factors to be dealt with in the science of disease is the chemical influence of the emotional activities of the being. Very few realize this fact.

It has been recognized for a long time, that joy, sorrow, etc., exercise a certain influence upon physical health; we know for instance, that when we can develop the right kind of emotional states, can stimulate the proper feelings, we will, by reason of the fact, be able to greatly improve the health of the patient, but it is not generally known that the emotional states actually generate chemical substances, which have the capacity of healing or poisoning the body. Yet, this is absolutely correct.

It should be borne in mind, that there is a certain rhythm appertaining to all emotional activity, a rhythm different from that of Mental activity, or Physical.

To make the matter a little clearer, we must understand that from the Kosmic Energy, Mind, Astral Light and Ether are alike generated; in other words, each of these substances is constituted by reason of the formation of a unit or ultimate atom, which is itself, a structure formed by the combination of a vast multitude of the atoms of the Kosmic Energy, or Buddhi. This combination causes the Unit or Ultimate Atom to move with a certain rhythm, or, in other words, on a certain octave. Now, all Atoms and Molecules moving on this octave, that is to say, the Astral or Desire Octave, become, by reason of that fact, Astral Fluid, or Desire Stuff, we might call it. This Desire Stuff is, therefore, moving on this octave and this is the material of which emotions are formed, that is to say, emotion is the activity of this principle; but it should be borne in mind, also, that all emotional activity when coming from thought, or whatever it may be, has the effect of moving on this rhythm and thus expressing itself through this substance, this Astral Fluid. The Astral Fluid is, therefore, drawn from the Astral

Plane, and also generated within the human aura by reason of the expression of Emotion, feeling at any time and under all circumstances.

Not only is this true, but there are two general classes of emotions, those which we term positive and others which are termed negative. Now we are not to understand by these expressions always exactly the same thing. In the more chemical sense or the physical sense we find that those positive emotions are the ones which move outward from the center; that is to say, the ones which have the effect of causing a wave of emotion to pass out through the Desire Body, moving outward from the center to the surface and thus acting upon the world without; the negative emotions are those, the tendency of which is to cause the wave to pass inward, so a vortex is thus formed and it is drawn through this fluid to the center, as it were, being an indrawing, a sucking motion, which draws inward from the world without.

These are the two emotions which may be briefly described as being Will and Desire. Whatever is operative from Desire will, therefore, make the person subject to outward influences, or become subjective, while all those emotions are positive, act from the center on the world without and thus become objective. The two may be described as being active and receptive in their character.

Each emotion, however, has a rate of vibration peculiar to itself, different from what every other has; that is to say, whenever an emotion is awakened within a being it causes the Astral Fluid to move in accordance with that particular rate of vibration pertaining to that specific emotion. The result is the rate of vibration in the Astral Body is continually changing; never is the same. It is always fluctuating in accordance with the diverse emotions which are active within the Desire Body. As are the emotions so will be the vibrations of the Desire Body at a given moment. Now, each of these rates of vibration not only expresses itself in this way and as the expression of a certain emotion, but it also expresses itself in form, color and sound, so that by looking at the Astral Body of a person you can tell, if you know how to interpret the colors, the emotions, which are moving within his being. Not only this, but you may also, if you are clairaudient, hear the sound which emanates from him, and thus ascertain the nature of those emotions; and not only can you do this, but you will see certain geometrical figures, which are continually forming in the Desire Body fluctuating back and forth, presenting a kaleidoscopic view before you. These geometrical figures, which are formed by the atoms of the Astral Fluid as they gather, continually changing according to the emotion, which is moving this force, form the crystals we will say, though of course, in the Astral form, of chemicals, which are just as definitely chemical as anything we meet with in the pharmacopoeia. The chemical is here generated through the emotion, and each specific rate of vibration, representative of each specific emotion, expresses itself in a chemical peculiar to itself.

These chemicals are thus generated and are manifesting themselves through the Astral Body. In the course of time, they descend until they influence the etheric double, and we have the corresponding chemical in the etheric double. At last, however, as this permeates every cell of the human body, this Etheric Chemical becomes physical in the grosser sense, assumes its more solid form, and thus we have a chemical accumulation in the cells of the body, corresponding to the Emotional Chemical, which was formed in the Astral Body.

As a matter of fact, the chemicals in the physical body are merely those Astral Chemicals on a lower octave, and are the perfect counterpart of the same. Some of these chemicals are benevolent and some malevolent. Those usually called positive are benevolent, that is, which are in accordance with the general processes of the human body, with the general state of the physical health. This is what is meant by the term "Positive Emotion," namely an emotion, the tendency of which, is to generate a chemical which is in itself beneficial to the human body.

On the other hand those Emotions are termed Negative, which generate a chemical, which descending into the physical body, will there deposit something which is detrimental to the health and life of the physical body.

Professor Elmer Gates has located some sixty-five of these chemicals by the stimulation of certain emotions in the hearts of people and having them exhale the breath into a glass tube and then analyzing this breath, which is left upon the sides of the tube, both before and after the emotions are stimulated and recognizing the differnce in the chemical constitution of the breath. Also, by examining the perspiration, which has been found to yield chemical precipitation, and by this chemical analysis, which has been repeated hundreds and thousands of times, it is now known that those emotions which produce very dangerous results, have dangerous effects on the physical health, which are known by physicians to have such without their knowing the reason why — are now known to be in their nature poisonous, to deposit a poison, which would have a corresponding effect if administered in the form of a drug.

Those emotions, therefore, which are detrimental, are so because they form a chemical substance, which in its nature, poisons the body. On the other hand, the curative emotions are such because they produce the very same chemicals, which would be used by an intelligent physician in treating the body.

It is, therefore, not a vague imaginary practice to employ certain emotional states to cure certain diseases, but it is simply a definite application of this law of Astral Chemistry and is, in fact, a matter of exact science, and has no basis of guesswork about it. There is nothing so scientific as the application of these emotional states.

It is now known that joy, hope, cheer, optimism, happiness, cheerfulness — all these diverse emotional states, laughter, mirth, wit, etc., have a beneficial effect on the body, as well as courage, determination, resolution, — everything of a positive character. On the other hand, sorrow, misery, despair, agony, hatred, jealousy and everything of that kind have a detrimental effect and are, consequently, termed Negative in their character. But why is this? Because these emotions generate certain chemicals, it has been said of old, "Joy doeth good like a medicine, but sorrow drieth up the bones." As a matter of fact, Sorrow in its activity generates a substance which cannot be detected from carbonate of lime and therefore, increases the lime in the bones, the mineral matter, which makes them dry, hard, and brittle, which produces the condition of old age, as it settles in the system. Joy, consequently, has the counteracting effect, it increases the animal matter and thus neutralizes the accumulation of lime, and perpetuates a state of youth.

Those emotions which are Saturnine in their character, that is to say, such as deal with Black Art, Magic, Sorcery, Occultism, etc., emotions accompanying those things and the use of those powers to do evil — the emotions which would accompany such an attitude of mind, generate lead, and are capable of lead poisoning.

The use of the Will, or the activity of the Will, generates iron, and is the sovereign remedy for improvished blood, where iron is lacking.

Sexual love generates copper, and it will be found to be there in great abundance, owing to this influence.

The activity of a continually changing emotional state, fluctuating from one state to another, continually changing, going up and down as the mind changes; the emotion, which is expressive of this changefulness will generate mercury.

A violent, quick temper, not given to hate, but rather that which flies from one extreme to another, will produce quicksilver.

Hatred, fiendish antagonism, or anything, in fact, which we express under the term of hate, where there is wish for evil to come to a person, where hate is expressed, will generate sulphur, and the system is liable to become poisoned under the influence of sulphur.

These chemicals are very often found in the body, when it is definitely known that no such chemical has been taken into the system physically. In fact, the body is composed of chemicals. It is well-known, that it is nothing but a chemical laboratory, but it is not so well-known, that the Astral Body is likewise, a laboratory of Astral Chemicals and those chemicals in the physical body, are simply the Astral Chemicals, descending, and manifesting on the physical plane. If you succeed in removing those Astral Chemicals, that is to say, changing them, changing the emotions so that those astral chemicals will cease to be produced, you can in time, change the chemicals of the

15

physical body, for the physical body is nothing in the world, but the production of the condition of the astral body on the physical plane. Remember, however, that it takes a little time for the astral chemicals to descend and manifest in the physical, consequently, simply changing the emotions will not cure a state of poisoning, which has already taken place in the body. By changing the emotions you simply cease to generate any more of those emotions and consequently the poisons no longer are formed, but all that are there in the astral body still remain unless you can bring a powerful influence to disorganize them, which is possible, but very difficult, — those remaining will descend to the Etheric Body, and ultimately to the Gross Physical Body, there generating those chemicals; consequently the treatment must go on until those astral, etheric and physical chemicals have been eliminated. But no treatment will be successful, which does not take notice of the fact, that all those poisons are the results of astral poisoning, growing out of emotional states because, if the old emotions continue to go on, if the person continues to be swayed by them, he will continue to generate those poisons without any cessation and consequently, he will have to continue to neutralize those poisons, and continue to have them cured and removed, because just as long as the poisoning goes on, just so long will there be a job for the doctor, and it will continue just as long as those emotions are continued. Consequently, there is no such thing as perfect health, until man has learned to feel properly, has learned to have the right kind of emotions; and this is the reason why the influence of certain religions, Christian Science, New Thought and others are very often so beneficial. It is because, they change the emotional state, and changing that emotional state, everything is found to be in a state of harmony, a state of health and peace.

Do not, therefore, for one moment, conceive that health is possible, excepting through an harmonious state of vibration — harmony with one's self, with God and the Universe. Dissatisfaction and everything inharmonious; discordant states of vibration, which do not make people good, indeed, can only express themselves in a state of physical discord, or physical poisoning, must be dealt with the same as any other kind of poisoning.

Improper emotional states, must, therefore, continue to poison the body just as long as they are endured or tolerated. When we have learned to bring about the proper emotional states the positive states, generally expressed under the term optimism, in place of the negative, detrimental, inharmonious, malevolent states, expressed under the term pessimism, generally those which are pessimistic toward others as well as toward ourselves — whenever we have done this and not before, will we displace the state of poisoning, resulting in ill health, with that state of harmony resulting in perfect health. Disease being the outgrowth of emotional poisoning, can be cured only by those particular states of emotion which develop those chemicals, which are the natural antidotes for those poisons.

Now, as every chemical, that ever is found in a poisoned body may be generated there through certain emotional states, it follows, that the fiction of the physician, that you have to have drugs to cure certain conditions is absolutely untrue. It is never necessary to administer drugs to the body in the physical form, because the emotions are quite capable of generating every chemical in the world, and will do so if the proper emotions are active.

The cure, therefore, for all those troubles is the CONTROL of the EMOTIONS; keeping them under proper guidance, so that we will feel the way we want to, we will have the emotions, which we realize we ought to have, and therefore, will generate the proper chemicals. If the physician can control the emotions of his patient, he can cure every disease from which the physical body may ever suffer.

L E S S O N   O N

F U N C T I O N A L   D I S E A S E S

When physicians get hold of a patient and cannot tell what is the matter with him, they say he lacks tone; the system must be toned up, yet there is not one of them who knows or pretends to know what he means by this expression, toning up his system and the lack of tone. This lack of tone, really represents a condition which is at the foundation of all diseases of this type which are so difficult to handle. Just what is meant by "Tone" is the question. As a matter of fact "tone" is the condition presented when all the functions of the body are being performed in the proper manner; the lack of "tone" is when a functional disturbance takes place.

Functional diseases are not to be confused with conditions where the body is astrally poisoned or anything of that kind. They have a specific place in pathology. We speak of heart disease, for instance, but as a matter of fact, we do not mean that the heart is diseased. Were anything to get wrong with the heart organically the patient would not last very long. What we mean by heart disease is a weakened or disturbed condition of the cardiac nerve center, which causes the heart to get out of gear in the sense that the proper quantity of nervous stimuli is not communicated to the heart. The result is, the heart is not able to perform its functions; thus we say it is diseased; that is, it is out of harmony, so with all the other diseases that are to be included under the functional head.

We should conceive of an organ or muscle as being a machine, a motor, in fact, or rather, a machine run by a motor. The nerve center controlling this organ or muscle is the motor that runs the machine. Now, the analogy is perfect between the nerve center and the motor in ordinary machines; if the motor receives a proper quantity of electricity it will run the machine in the proper manner. If it does not receive a sufficient quantity, the force will be weak, and consequently, the machine will run at a very low pressure. The more electricity the motor receives, the higher will be the pressure at which the machine will be run. If the current becomes too strong, the pressure will become too high and the machine will be over run, or rather, will run to pieces.

If the current is not steady, but is disturbed, of course, the action of the motor will be disturbed.

The great problem, therefore, is to preserve the equilibrium in the electrical current running to the motor; so that the machine will be run properly. Wires connect the motor with the dynamo where the electrical current is generated, consequently, if anything gets wrong with the wires the motor will not get the proper current, or if the dynamo is not being run properly.

Now, in applying those principles to health, the motor, or nerve center if it receive the proper quantity of Prana, will act in the proper manner. By reason of this stimulation, it will carry on the organ, causing it to perform its proper function. If the current becomes too weak, then the activity of the nerve center will be correspondingly weakened. If the current becomes too strong the pressure will be too high; there will be an over activity of the organ; or if the currents be interrupted, broken, then we will see a spasmodic activity of the organ as in the case of palpitation of the heart followed by a depression.

The nerves are the live wires which convey the Prana to the nerve center and if the proper quantity of Prana — and not too much — be communicated along these nerves to the nerve center, it will act normally; if too much, then abnormally.

The dynamo which directs all the Prana going to the functional nervous system is so far as the physical is concerned, the Solar Plexus and Sympathetic Nervous System being closely identified with the functional state of health.

But the point you should bear in mind is this: If the current of nervous stimuli flowing over the sympathetic nervous system and reaching the nerve centers governing those organs, be normal, if the equilibrium be maintained, perfect health in those functions will be the result; each nerve center will receive a sufficient quantity of Prana to enable it to compel the organ to perform its proper functions. But if the current be weak or too strong or spasmodic a corresponding result will take place.

Functional diseases then, are simply cases of low vitality; too much stimulation or a weak circulation of the vital force. They are not to be treated in any other way excepting in and through the regulation of the circulation of the nerve force. If you can control this, you can cure any functional disease in the world, no matter what it may be.

The question, then, for the physician to solve is HOW to control the Circulation of this Vital Force. There is no other cure for functional diseases, and this will cure in every instance. If physicians would only realize that functional diseases are due to a low state or an improper circulation of the vital principle and not due to a lack of any chemicals in the system or to the presence of any chemicals, if, in a word, they would treat functional diseases biologically rather than chemically, we would have no trouble in the treatment of those diseases.

But the question is, why is the circulation of the vital force irregular? What is the cause of this disturbance in the equilibrium? Why does it not always circulate regularly, equilibrimatically? Why is it that this discordant condition takes place at all? This matter is made clear when you realize that the Prana which is the life principle or force which circulates through the nerves, is operative in and through the Astral Body; that is to say, the currents of Prana run through the Astral Body. As these pranic currents are passing through the desire stuff it follows they must be influenced largely by the circulation of the desire principle. As the movement of the Desire Body is, so will be the movement of the Prana, that is to say, the Desire Body is its constituent principle, moves along a certain line, takes a certain channel, and the result is, it carries with it quite a quantity of Prana, consequently, the circulation of the Prana is governed by the circulation of the Desire Body. As the Desire Body circulates in accordance with the emotions, every movement in the Astral being the effect of a corresponding emotional state, it follows that the direction of the circulation in the Prana depends upon the emotional activities.

Those emotional activities, being dependent upon the particular nature of the emotion, upon each specific emotion, it is, therefore, seen that the entire circulation of the Life Force is absolutely the effect of the emotions of the individual. A man suffering from a functional disease is suffering from it because of the discordant character of his emotions; because they are not under his control, but are moving in an improper manner. If the circulation be spasmodic it indicates that his emotions are spasmodic, they are flighty, there is nothing steady, nothing continuous in the emotional state. If the current be too strong and if it be too strong all over the body — generally speaking, if there be an over-stimulated condition, it is because the person is excitable, passionate, and his emotions are always at a fever heat. At any time when this condition is present, it indicates a fever heat of emotions. If, on the contrary, the system is weakened and there is a very low state of vitality, it will generally indicate Ipseal emotions; everything is self-relative; he is thinking of self all the time, and that draws the Prana inward, the result being that there is none left to stimulate the activities of the bodily organs.

But usually these functional troubles manifest in the form of a lack of balance in the vitalization of the diverse parts of the body; that is to say, one organ is well stimulated; another is starving. It is not because there is not a sufficient quantity of vitality, but the balance, the equilibrium, is not preserved. It is not more vitality that is required but rather a proper distribution of the vital force.

Now, when you realize that every class of emotions is related to different organs of the body, just as the different parts of the body are related to the mind, the different parts of the brain and different kinds of thought — there are certain parts of the body, however, that are specifically related to corresponding emotional states — consequently those emotions will stimulate, corresponding nerve centers; at the same time they will draw the nerve force away from other nerve centers. Just as sure as those emotions are persisted in, they will thus starve the system of the blood which it requires. The student should, for this reason endeavor to ascertain, in a given case what the emotional states are which are at fault. He can discover this by a little examination. See the disturbed condition, find out just what it is; what nerve centers are weak and what are over stimulated and then notice the different emotional states and see, as nearly as possible, what the physical effect is of the different emotional states of the patient. In time he will be enabled to diagnose the case emotionally, that is to find out the emotion that is at fault. Then try to restrain this emotion, to stimulate one that will have a counteracting effect; that is one that will stimulate the weakened nerve center and restrain the over-stimulated one. When the equilibrium in the emotional activity is established it will always result in a corresponding equilibrium of the vital circulation. Given this equilibrium, we will have the cure of all functional diseases, and they cannot be permanently cured otherwise.

It is for this reason that those healing cults which appeal to the emotions, with the object of establishing a state of emotional equilibrium — to always maintain the state of poise, balance, self-centeredness — where there can be no disturbance, have the effect which they have. They would be of no practical value were it not for this influence which they exercise upon the Desire Body, and consequently upon the circulation of the nerve force or Prana.

Any method which will restore the equilibrium in the circulation of the nerve force will cure any functional disease in the world. You may benefit the condition by applying nervous stimuli direct to the nerve center controlling the organ. Magnetic Healing and the other metaphysical healing methods have, therefore, been found of very much value in the treatment of functional diseases, because they give the nerve force which that nerve center is starving. Giving this nerve force, they establish the equilibrium, they strengthen the organ or rather the nerve center, so that it makes the organ perform its proper functions.

Likewise, Suggestive Therapeutics is of great value because it regulates the circulation of the nerve force and this sends that force to the nerve center, enabling it to compel the organ to perform its proper function.

The only value of any treatment employed by the physician, then, for functional diseases is in its ability to stimulate the vital force in those centers. There may be various methods of doing this. There may be different causes which lead up to this disturbance of the nervous circulation, as, for instance, pressure of the vertebrae upon some of the nerves. However, this does not effect the organ, because it is not the cerebro-spinal nerves so much that lead to them, but the sympathetic nerves; but the bones may press upon some of the nerves. In that case it requires the work of an osteopath, or a chiropractor to relieve the pressure, but it is simply the application of the same principle; or in increasing the circulation in certain muscles, mechano-therapy, applied in the form of manipulation, will increase the circulation of the nerve force and consequently, will relieve the trouble.

But bear in mind that in all those methods the thing that CURES is the equilibrium in the circulation of the nerve force in the nerve center. The method that is employed is simply a means of bringing about this change in the circulatory proportion of the vital force. Realizing this, the treatment, therefore, should be anything that will lead up to the accomplishment of this equilibrium in the circulatory activity of the Prana. That method which will most easily lead unto this result is the best, under the circumstances.

There is no disease of a functional character to which flesh is heir, that cannot be cured by this method and cured with comparative ease. There is no functional disease that can be cured permanently in any other way. Even those medicines such as arsenic and cactina that are given by physicians, are really given for the purpose of accomplishing this result, by causing a certain stimulus to be imparted to the nerve centers in an artificial manner which will thus draw to them the nervous force.

Remember, therefore, that in our method of healing we are employing the same fundamental principle that all intelligent physicians employ. Our methods are, of course, a little more scientific, they are more fundamental than theirs, but it is not a new departure, it is not a new fad, it is simply the application of the old physiological method of removing the cause and allowing Nature to take care of itself.

L E S S O N   O N

M E N T A L   C H E M I S T R Y

The Astral Vibrations are really nothing more than duplicates
of the Astral Octave of vibrations which have already taken place on the
Mental Octave. The Astral Plane is but the reflection of the Mental
Plane. Nothing ever takes place there until after it has taken place on
the Mental Plane. The result is such vibration as it operates through
the Manas, expresses itself on the next lower octave, or the Astral, thus
producing an emotion corresponding to it.

All our emotions are, consequently, but the duplication of our
thoughts. No thought is ever generated in the mind but what sooner or
later is duplicated in the heart. Of course, the emotional duplicate
may be much more powerful in one case than it is in another, but our
emotions are the effects of our thinking.

Having realized the influence of the emotions on the health both
in reference to the directing of the Life Force and thus the cure of
functional diseases or their cause in either case, and also to the gen-
eration of chemical substances which poison — when we realize that all
this emotional activity is but the effect of the thought, we can readily
see the importance of thought control. The statement, "As a man thinketh
in his heart, so is he," is absolutely true; that is, as a man thinks in
his emotions, the emotion being the effect of thought. Now as man's
thought descends to the Mental Octave and generates corresponding emotions, so the man becomes, that is, so his entire character is made up
and every thing of the kind.

The point we want you to notice is this: the activities of the
heart are emotional expressions, are not self-generative, but are the
effects of thought vibrations, and each thought sets up a vibratory force
in the Mental Body, which will, in time, descend to the Astral vehicle
and set up in the Astral substance a corresponding emotion. It is not
simply that thought generates emotion, but each specific thought generates a thing in harmony with itself, and also thoughts are divided into

positive and negative, corresponding to the positive and negative emotional states. In fact our emotions of fear are the outgrowth in the Desire Body of a belief in danger. Were it not for a previous thought of danger, there would be no emotion of fear and it is always the outgrowth of our opinion about things, about their nature, that is expressed in fear, horror, anger, resentment, and all those emotional states. It is likewise, the thought of one's self as being inferior or subordinate to another, as being dependent upon another, upon outside influences, etc. which manifests itself in fear of those objects and in emotions which move inward from the surface. A thought which is self-expressive, which makes the self the center and its positive outflowing in its attitude, will necessarily produce positive emotions, which will have the same influence.

It is not necessary to go into details here. All that is necessary is for the pupil to bear in mind that the emotions are the shadows, the reflections of corresponding thoughts on the Mental Octave, and must always respond to the nature of that thought no matter what it may be.

Man's attitude of mind and feeling has a very great deal to do with the state of his health. In fact, when we realize that the Astral Body, controlled by the thinking, is in fact, the expresssion of thought on the Astral Octave, and that it controls the circulation of the Prana, and therefore, the conditions of functional diseases, vitality, etc., and also generates all the chemical combinations which are found in the body, we can readily see how terribly important the character of our thinking is in reference to the treatment of disease.

It should also be borne in mind that our own thought determines our positive and negative relation to the universal thought. All the thoughts which others have thought are drawn to us when we become negatively polarized with them. In fact, we are at all times more or less influenced by the thoughts of others, it being utterly impossible for one to entirely disconnect himself from the thought of others individually and collectively. In fact, thought which has been generated in all past ages is still there and is drawn to us to a greater or less extent. The more we harmonize with this thought, being negatively polarized, the more thought we draw to us.

Diseases which are the outgrowth of popular thinking are very likely to be drawn to one who is under those influences.

It should, likewise, be borne in mind, that there are forces in nature which are vibratively harmonious with those thoughts and thus by maintaining this attitude of mental vibratory harmony, we draw those forces to us. The result is a disease which has been generated by thought vibrations of a certain kind, expressing themselves through emotional vibrations of the same rate, will also have that rate of vibration, for it must be borne in mind that disease is not simply a subjective condition; it is really a form of energy which has been generated

24

in the physical body by reason of this discordant state of vibration. It is a kind of spiritual virus, so to speak, which is present in the Desire Body. Now, this poison, this Septic Ether, continues to move with the same rate of vibration as the Diseased Mind and Astral Force move with. It is in fact, the physical aspect, that is to say the Etheric aspect of that same force, that same Astral vibration. Now, if one is thinking thoughts which have the same vibration, he is polarized with the disease. If he becomes negative, he will naturally draw it to him, becoming the negative pole, and thus contract it.

It is largely due to the fact that man's thought is diseased, that he is drawing to him the disease influence of those around him. There would be practically little danger in times of epidemics if people were perfectly pure and spiritual in their thinking, if there were nothing in their thinking which was in harmony with the epidemic, because in a majority of cases, epidemics are a diseased influence, that is a discordant, inharmonious influence which has been generated through the improper thinking and feeling of the public. It is terrible to contemplate, nevertheless, it is true that epidemics of vice are just as prevalent as epidemics of disease. These epidemics of vice come about and go from mind to mind, and usually they are followed by epidemics of disease. In fact, these epidemics of impure thought, followed by impure emotions and lastly by impure action, must also be followed by improper states of health and disease. When we realize this we can then see what a terrible thing it is to follow habits of discordant thought.

Bear in mind that each phase of discordant thought, that is each type of mental discord, manifests itself ultimately in a corresponding type of physical discord or disease. If one at the same time be negative, whether he has this particular type of thought or not, if he be negative, he is likely to draw it to him, and this is why in time of epidemics there is so much danger in fear, fear representing that attitude of mind which makes the Mental Body of man negative; which causes it to draw the currents inward from the surface, with the result that vortexes are formed which will allow the entrance of forces from the outside. Thus the person opens the door for the entrance of all those influences. There is a story of a man, in the Orient, meeting the Spirit of Cholera and he asks him who he is. He says, "I am the Death. I came from Damascus; fifty thousand died there; I killed five thousand and Fear killed the rest." And this is really true. The fear of people has the tendency to draw the force of disease to them when it would not come otherwise; that is, it opens the way, makes them respond to the influence.

Now, it is because of this fact, that the cities are so unhealthy. It is not because of improper sanitation, because of the dirt and those things, although they are bad enough, — it is not from physical causes that cities are so much more unhealthful than the country. It is because

25

the general mind, the public mind is there so much more powerful in its suggestive influence, than it is in the country. In the country districts, man is able to preserve his integrity of thought much better than he is in the crowded cities, because the mind of the crowd not being anything like as powerful there as it is in the cities. It is practically impossible for a man in the densely populated city to preserve anything resembling integrity of thought. He must submit to the mind of the crowd, and therefore, he is influenced, — he is dragged down to that level. Also in uninhabited localities it is found much better, and much more conducive to health and everything of the kind because more conducive to individuality of thought to live in those out of the way places, than even in the country where there are very many neighbors, because in this way you escape the mental environment and are able to establish one of your own.

Further, it should be borne in mind that as thought vibrations move, each moving in accordance with its own particular rate of vibration, the lower rates of vibration stay close to the earth. There is an attraction between them and the earth. It is only the thoughts which have a correspondingly high rate of vibration that are able to rise to a high elevation and as they rise to this high elevation, they are thus liberated from all contact with those below and cannot easily be drawn down to the grade generally vibrating very low in their thinking. The result is that those higher vibrations, that is, those high in the sense of being more elevated physically, are more removed from the psychology of the crowd, consequently less liable to generate diseases.

It will be found that they will also have less power to determine the direction of one's thinking, thus enabling him to attain a great deal higher degree of individuality of thought than he could otherwise. It is for this reason that high elevations, the tops of mountains, have been from time immemorial, the favorite resort of recluses and thinkers, philosophers and mystics who have sought to get away from the spirit of the crowd, because they are there able to think clearly, to think as they want to think instead of being dominated by the lower influences. As we thus rise upward, we get above the thoughts of the crowd, and are, therefore, not dominated by them and do not, as a result, draw to us those influences, of a physical and astral character, which correspond to the thoughts of the crowd.

It will, therefore, be seen that it will be much better for sanitariums and hospitals to be placed on the tops of mountains, than to be placed in the crowded cities or down low. By placing them there, the patients will be brought out of the lower thought atmosphere and thus will be able to get free from those disease influences. It is true, on the other hand, that if one wants to be of great service he may live in the crowd, in the cities, on the lower elevations and thus, by thinking the highest that he can, help to purify and elevate the thought atmosphere of the world and in this way make it easier for others to maintain a higher elevation of thought than otherwise they could.

Thought vibration is really the principle that governs Emotional Vibration, therefore, all diseased conditions that manifest in the human body are directly or indirectly the effect of emotional states engendered by thought vibrations which are, in turn, the effects of mental attitude. There is no greater error than the idea that disease can be cured permanently without changing a man's opinions. The idea that a change of religious belief, philosophical belief, etc. will bring about a change in man's physical condition is absolutely correct. The fact which has been so often noticed by modern students, that the acquiring of a belief in New Thought, Spiritualism, any of those cults which has brought about a radical change in the mental view point has been accompanied by an improvement in health, is absolutely true. The general belief establishes a certain mean Thought Vibration, it establishes a certain type of thinking, which is all of that general vibratory type. The result is, a typical vibration is established, which, in turn, manifests itself in a typical Astral condition eventuating in typical physical vibratory states, which produce chemicals of that particular type. The result is, man's physical condition is, in the last analysis, the effect of his beliefs, of his creed, so to speak. Where a man really believes a creed, and is sincere in it, that creed establishes his state of health. A man who is pessimistic must necessarily become a hypochondriac, in every instance, it cannot fail. The man who has a belief that all the people in the world are sinners and are going to hell and everything of that kind, who acts from a pessimistic view of humanity, is sure to get bilious, and it affects him all the way through. We find it stated that Robespierre became so bilious, as a result of his conducting the French Revolution during the Reign of Terror, that his stomach would not digest anything but oranges; he had to live exclusively on a diet of oranges, because they were the only thing that would counteract the bile which was continually generating in his system by reason of his line of thinking. Many people have been sick all their lives because of the disease conditions that were generated by their beliefs. It is utterly useless for a person to argue to us that the old orthodox Calvinists ever had good health; they were bound to be bilious or hypochondriacal, one of the two. The feeling of jealousy must generate a jaundiced condition, always. On the other hand when a person becomes optimistic, the circulation of the blood is stimulated and it has the tendency to cure most of his disease. Optimism is a splendid antidote for nearly all diseases. It is not that pessimism is wrong morally so much as that it generates a certain type of vibrations which express themselves in corresponding physical conditions that poison the system. When one, therefore, who has taken an unhappy point of view, changes his philosophy, his religion, he begins a new form of thought vibration which stimulates corresponding emotions and generates new chemicals, and those become naturally an antidote for those chemicals that were generated in the system of his former belief. Consequently he is almost sure to improve for a period of time, at least, after his change of thought, though after a while he may establish a new system of poisoning, when he will need another change in order to transform his vibration and thus change the chemical combination of his being.

It is for this reason that the crystallization of thought is not good for the health, whatever it may be for the philosophy; it is not good for the health, it is better that there should be a continual process of change, a transformation of thought going on all the time. Nothing is so disastrous as fossilizing of the mental senses. Instead of this, we should try to grow and expand, and transform our thought. Our minds, in fact, should be in a state of flux, so that we are going through this transformation all the time. In this way our vibration will continually be changing; the chemical combinations will go through a state of transformation; instead of the body being a pharmacy or a chemical establishment, it will become an Alchemical Laboratory where there will be continual transformations and that is really the foundation of health — continuous change. This is possible only by a vital, living, transforming mental attitude, which is continuously expressing itself in new thoughts, and therefore, new emotions which lastly express themselves in new vibratory conditions giving rise to new chemicals, and therefore, building up a new body. As the body is thus continually renewed, is giving way to new conditions, going through new transformations, perfect health is the result. Disease grows up as a result of stagnation which, therefore, must be overcome by originality of thought, by a continuous changing of the thought and thus the Desire. As the Thought Vibration is, so will the Emotional Vibration be, and as is the Emotional Vibration, so will be the chemical combinations which are formed in the physical body, and as these chemicals are, so will be the state of physical health. Likewise, as is the emotional vibrations, so will be the circulation of the Life Force, therefore, so will be the state of functional health throughout the system.

There can, therefore, be no permanent healing of the body and no permanent establishment of a correct emotional state excepting by a change in the intellectual view point, a change in the man's thinking. It is, therefore, necessary that we should entirely transform the point of view, the philosophy and the religion of a man in order to heal his body permanently.

Disease is the natural effect of sin; not simply sin which is expressed in outward emotions, but sinful emotion and sinful thinking; that is, incorrect and erroneous thinking, and consequently man must learn to think correctly, truly and in harmony with unity. When he has learned integrity and unity of thought, when he has learned to think in the Cosmos instead of a Chaos, and has learned to practice that higher principle of thinking in harmony with Divine Law, he will then generate the correct emotions which will establish correct vibratory states, resulting in correct chemical forms in his body. This habit of correct thinking will express itself in a perfect physical condition. When he quits sinning mentally, he will quit suffering the consequences of this mental sin. He will cease to draw to himself disease, and will sow in his system health, because he will think healthfully, rationally and justly.

We can never permanently heal the body except by healing the mind, except by bringing the mind into a state of Cosmic Order in harmony with Divine Law. When this is accomplished, we will have accomplished the perfect health of the body. It does not require any medicine to cure a man when he has ceased to sin in his thinking. Health will be the natural consequence of proper normal and harmonious thought. "As a man thinketh, so is he;" that is to say, so he becomes, because all the lower principles of his being are nothing but the effects of his thinking.

LESSON ON

MENTAL PICTURING

The force which directs the vibrative forces throughout the
system is MENTAL PICTURING. Form, color and sound being inseparably
connected with all vibratory manifestation, it follows that whenever a
certain rate of vibration is established within the auric forces, it
manifests itself through the formation of forms, or figures in that
energy corresponding to the pictures, likewise in certain colors,
shades and tints and also in corresponding colors.

The point that the student should bear in mind is this: Whenever the energy begins to move in accordance with a certain rate of
vibration, immediately that energy, by reason of that vibration,
gathers into certain geometrical figures, corresponding to that rate
of vibration, each figure being the effect of that vibratory state.
These organisms are formed just as distinctly as any organisms on the
physical plane, these geometrical figures being the organs of all
chemical formations. Likewise, the colors and the sounds are produced
and these are all the effects of corresponding rates of vibration; the
rate of vibration must necessarily express itself in this form, color
and sound. Inasmuch as the vibration expresses itself in this way, it
should be borne in mind that by visualizing the consciousness upon a
given form, color, or sound so that there is repeated in our consciousness the vibration corresponding to that, that form, color or sound is
set up within the aura. If it be a clear mental perception or rather mental
picture, that is to say, a picture of an intellectual character, it
will set up that vibration in the Mental Body. If it be emotional rather,
it follows that it is established in the Astral Fluid. In either case,
however, we have the vibration springing from the picture.

It has been shown in previous lessons that vibration is the force
back of the different states of health and disease, in fact, health
being merely an harmonious state of vibration, while disease is a discordant vibratory state, and it was also shown that chemical formations

30

were produced through vibrations in the mental body, for Mental Chemistry is nothing but the effect through the chemistry of the form which is generated through the vibration passing through the Mental Body. Astral Chemistry is also the organisms which are produced in the Astral Body by reason of the vibration imparted to the Astral Fluid. The emotion, therefore, generates the form, the geometrical figure which is the product of this vibratory activity. Thus all of the vibrations which act upon either the Astral or the Mental Body, and through the Astral, upon the life force, that which also acts upon the Etheric Double — in fact, that vibratory force which is the law back of the manifestations in the three worlds, is the effect of Mental Picturing, by the picture which is formed in mind or the idea, in other words, the vibration is established. The moment we form in mind the picture, or the idea, we set up the corresponding vibration. As we are negative, drawing into the center, being governed by Desire, we cause this motion, this vibratory impulse arising from the idea, to flow inward, from the surface to the center, and as we are positive, as we are acting through the Will, we cause, through the fiat this vibration to move outward from the center of our being to the surface. This vibration is the outgrowth of Mental Picturing, the first step from the picture, Will, being the positive expression of this vibration, causing it to flow outward from the center, while Desire becomes the Negative expression and causes it to flow inward from the surface toward the center. These twofold activities, inward from the surface to the center, or Desire, and outward from the center to the surface, or Will, are the twofold activities of Mental Picturing. Mental Picturing, however, is the principle back of vibration, which expresses itself in and through vibration. Everything, therefore, is the outgrowth of Mental Picturing.

In order, therefore, to accomplish any results which we would wish to accomplish in our bodies, it is only necessary to establish the requisite vibration. If we can control the vibratory activity of the aura, we can in this way, control the state of health, the chemicals that are formed in the aura, the circulation of the different principles and everything of the kind, because the state or condition of all those principles is the effect of the rate of vibration which is going on within the aura. Consequently, to control the vibration is to control the harmony or discord as the case may be, which is the cause of health and disease. It is also to regulate the formation of chemicals and everything of the kind.

It will be readily seen that control of the vibration of the aura gives control of the entire physical, astral and mental condition of the being and as this vibration is the direct result of the mental picturing, of the pictures that are specifically formed in the consciousness, it will follow that the control of those pictures gives a control of the entire system, because it controls the vibration. It is the func-

31

tion of the imagination to form those pictures. Of course, in the strictest sense of the word, the pictures formed by the imagination are Astral quite as much as they are mental; but the imagination deals with the formation of pictures — images — and it is thus its function to regulate the imagination, the visualizing upon certain things, and as we control the visualizing, we secure a control of the vibration as it goes on throughout the entire system. It is for this reason that control of the imagination is so very important. The difficulty is, so many people do not realize that the imagination is always directing vibration. They are willing to agree that a person can form mental pictures by concentration, by direct, systematic visualization, of course, he can form those pictures, but to their minds, it is not true that he is forming those pictures anyhow.

Now, this is the point which the student should bear in mind very carefully and persistently: You cannot keep from forming those pictures as you are allowing your imagination to operate, for all imaginary activity is imaging, is painting pictures in the consciousness and such visualization is directing the vibration of the Aura, is thus exercising its influence on the Astral and Mental Bodies and the Etheric Double. Thus the whole system is the product of the imagination, little as people are willing to realize it.

It is as true today as it was in Napoleon's time, that imagination rules the world, for every thought and every emotion is really the outgrowth of imagination. The vibratory forces which move throughout the system, which build up those chemicals in the Mental Body, the Astral Body and the Etheric Double, are the result of corresponding pictures which are the product of the imagination.

Do not for one moment be deceived. There is no force in your nature so potent for weal or woe as your own imagination. The Imagination should, therefore, be kept under control. You should use it for the purpose of forming mental pictures to direct the vibration in the proper manner. By this we mean that you should lay down in your mind a general field of vibration; you should realize the vibratory forces which you want to maintain; that is to say, realizing what effect you want to produce and the pictures necessary to generate the vibration which will produce that effect, and keep them always before the consciousness, by holding before you the picture. Keep imaging that result; continually keep visualizing upon it and in this way; by this process of visualization, keep the vibration going which will bring about that result.

It is really as a means unto the end of maintaining these pictures in mind that Healers have adopted the use of affirmations and denials. Denials, however, will be seen to be very undesirable when we realize that the power of everything of this kind consists in its ability for the formation of mental pictures, because denying a thing is just as efficacious for forming a picture of it as affirming. It is not what you say about a certain condition that directs the vibration; it is the fact that you have in your consciousness a picture of that condition, consequently, denials should never be resorted to because they simply help to fix in the subconscious a picture of the undesirable condition, and therefore, set up the vibration which will bring about the realization of that state. Affirmations, however, work along constructive lines, for by the affirmation we form a picture of the thing affirmed, and that is the end and aim of affirmations.

Suggestion is resorted to for precisely the same reason, and the only value in suggestion is in its utility as a means of forming a picture in the patient's mind of the desired condition.

Christian Science works along the same lines; its methods are simply directed unto the formation of the picture of health.

Banish the picture of disease, whatever it may be and establish the picture of health, and by so doing you are establishing the vibration of harmony in place of that of discord, and therefore, bringing about a state of health.

The healer in order to heal, must establish the vibration of harmony throughout his system, by the formation of the picture of health, and then transmit this harmonious vibration to the body of the patient. So, as a matter of fact, Mental Picturing is the force back of vibration and vibration the influence which heals.

There is no greater force in all the world than this force of mental picturing and it should be used as a means unto the end of bringing about health. However, it is not confined to therapeutics, but may be used for any kind of development. We may use it in the line of psychic development or for psychological unfoldment or anything of the kind. It is not, however, the key to the entire problem of human evolution. The Bible says, "As a man thinketh in his heart, so is he," and why? The thought of the heart as it descends to the man is an effect of the picture which is formed in the consciousness and thus, as in the picture, so will be the vibration, therefore, so will be the activity of the diverse principles of the being; so will be the vibratory force which will build up the being, along those lines.

We are the product of our ideals, because the ideals fix and determine the picture, hence the vibration and, therefore, the activity of the entire being. The value of the social or public ideals consists in its utility as a means of fixing a certain picture in the minds of the multitude. The public at large has the picture fixed in its consciousness; this picture is governing all its activities, governing its thinking and feeling, its physical, moral and mental states are the natural outgrowth of that picture, which is, in turn, the effect of the ideal.

Our ideals, therefore, make us. Civilization is the effect of our Utopias, because those Utopias determine the pictures which are

built up before us, and therefore, the vibration which shall pass
through our principles, which determine the formation of their chemicals and build up our being.

Visualization upon the picture is, therefore, the force back of
vibration. Everything which is accomplished through vibration is the
effect of this imaging. The imagination, being the imaging faculty,
is the creative faculty of the human consciousness. Imagination being creative, we become what we imagine. No matter whether we intend
it as constructive imagination or not, we are, nevertheless the effect
of our imagination. All development is the process of the "Ever becoming." We are everlastingly becoming what we imagine, not what we
imagine ourselves to be, simply, but whatever the imagination may be.
Whatever comes into our imagination, whatever picture is formed establishes the rate of vibration corresponding to itself and this in time
builds up, in the finer principles of our being a corresponding state.
Thus our very being is the effect of our imagination and we cannot in
any way escape the consequence. The only way is to hang up a new set of
pictures in our Mental Picture Gallery. If we do this, we will, in time
establish different vibrations, having different influences.

The thing to be borne in mind is that imagination does not simply
regulate the human character, the memory and those things, but it really
governs the formation, the organism of the body and of the constitution of man himself.

Imagination is not simply a moral force, but is also chemical,
its influence being quite as effective in the realm of Chemistry as any
of the other influences.

And so as are the pictures which we hang up in the Picture Gallery
of our Mind, so will be the vibration of our Aura and as is the vibration
of the Aura, so will be the chemical processes of the Mental and Astral
bodies and of the Etheric Double, and as are the processes of chemical
formation in those principles, so will be the chemical state of the
body, and as is this chemical state, and the vibration, the harmony
throughout the system, so will be the state of health or disease throughout the entire being.

LESSON ON

URIC ACID DISEASES

One particular type of diseases is due to the presence of Uric Acid in the Blood. The poison growing out of this condition or rather the effect of this poison in the blood, produces quite a number of diseases such as Rheumatism, Eczema, Scrofula when not caused by syphilis or mercurial poisoning, bright's disease and all of that type.

These diseases are simply the effects of Uric Acid in the blood and tissue. Of course, while it is simply in the blood it does not produce this disease effect, but it is the effort of Nature to throw off the uric acid poison, which produces the disease.

Understand, these diseases are simply curative attempts on the part of nature to accomplish relief. The body becomes diseased in this way.

What is the cause of Uric Acid getting in the blood? What is Uric Acid? It is an acid poison that accumulates in the system as a result of too much cooked protein. It is due to this and nothing else. The system requires a certain quantity of protein in order that the muscles and tissues may be built up, protein being the great tissue builder; but when this quantity has been supplied, when the tissues have been nourished with a sufficient quantity of protein, a sufficient quantity placed in the system, and the quantity placed in the system has continually increased until the tissues can make use of no more, until the maximum amount of nutrition has taken place and no more protein can be used by the system, if we continue to feed it, a fermentation takes place and the residue becomes transmuted into Uric Acid. Uric Acid is, therefore, the result of the fermentation of the surplus protein that has accumulated in the system. This Uric Acid accumulates in the blood and there remains in the form of an Ursal poison.

It is the mission of the kidneys to separate the Uric Acid from the blood and they will do this to the full extent of their ability. When the kidneys become overworked it is because there is too much work

for them to do. Bright's disease and all kidney troubles of that type
are due to an overworked condition of the kidneys and to the fact that
the kidney itself becomes poisoned, diseased, and the uric acid begins
to destroy the tissue of the kidney. It is for this reason that Bright's
disease is so difficult to cure. It is not, like the other uric acid
diseases, merely an effect of the poisoning of the system, but it is due
to the destruction of the kidney itself, and of course, as the kidney
is destroyed, its efficiency as a cleanser, as a separator is destroyed
and thus the poison gets worse and worse. Death is inevitable unless it
can be cured at a very early stage.

The other diseases are due to a poisoning of the tissue; that is
to say, scrofula and eczema are. Rheumatism is due to the accumulation
of uric acid in the joints, in the case of chronic rheumatism and in the
muscles in the case of inflammatory rheumatism. When it accumulates in
the muscles, the muscle becomes inflamed and this produces that acute
painful condition.

But these are all efforts at the purification of the blood. Those
medicines which are found to be most efficacious in the cure of those
uric acid diseases owe their curative properties to their utility as
stimulants of the kidneys, as by stimulating the kidneys, they help
them to throw off a greater quantity of the uric acid, while other
remedies are also advantageous in that they drive it out through the
skin. Anything which will quicken the excretory functions will be found
to be advantageous, to a certain extent, but the kidneys must do the
principal part of the work because it is their function to separate the
uric acid from the blood.

When one eats raw protein it will not cause this uric acid formation because it will not be digested. The System will not digest any
more raw protein than is required, it becoming difficult to digest it
in proportion to the quantity that is eaten, therefore, over-eating
will not do any serious harm if it be a raw food diet; but if the food be
cooked it becomes easy to digest and as a result of this ease of digestion we find that the system takes up too much of the food; it goes into
the blood and enters the tissue and thus produces the poison condition.
Of course, all meats have this tendency because they are all eaten cooked
and will be found to be very injurious. Beans, peas, lentils, in fact all
the legumens, are very detrimental for the same reason. Cheese is also
detrimental because it is made by applying heat to the milk, and boiled
milk, nut preparations made by heating are also detrimental. Peanut
butter unless made raw, is also detrimental because it imparts too much
cooked protein. The protein contained in cereals is also detrimental
to the health of the system, has a tendency to impart too much uric acid
to the system. All nuts in the cooked form, in fact, everything containing protein, if cooked will help to increase the quantity of Uric Acid.

In order to treat a patient who has any of those diseases it will, therefore, be found necessary first to stop him from eating cooked protein in order that he may not accumulate any more of this protein element. Therefore, whole grain bread if cooked, should be entirely excluded from his food. Put him on a diet of white bread if he is eating cooked bread. Do not allow him to eat any cheese, or any nut preparation made with fire, any parched nuts or nuts cooked in any way, meat, the legumens or anything of that kind; and also it will be found advantageous to entirely exclude from his diet all protein, for the time being, because the system is now loaded up with protein. This disease would not have come on had it not been that there was too much protein, and for a short time it is better to cut the patient off from those things, giving him a diet composed exclusively of sugar, starch foods, the organic salts, etc.

Also it must be borne in mind that the protein when taken in too large quantities does not stay in the system long, but is soon fermented and becomes uric acid, therefore, the abstaining from any protein should be for a few weeks at most; then begin to give the patient a diet of raw protein with the other foods.

But the uric acid must not only be kept out of the system, that is, we must not only cease to put the cooked protein into the system so as to make more uric acid, but we must get rid of that which is already in the system, therefore, a mere refraining from improper diet will not, alone, cure those diseases. We must get rid of the uric acid, and this is accomplished by nature, through the agency of the eliminant salts. These salts are potassium, sodium, calcium, magnesium, phosphorus, and silicon; but the inorganic salt is not an eliminant, only the organic salt; that is the salt where the molecules are bound together in loose affinity. They eliminate the poisons in this way; a molecule of sodium is united in loose affinity to another combination. You will find sodium and chloral united, forming sodium chloride in close affinity. To this compound molecule of sodium chloride there will be joined in loose affinity a molecule of sodium. When a molecule of some poisonous gas or acid comes in the vicinity of this sodium chloride as it has a strong affinity, a close affinity for sodium, the sodium leaves its loose affinity and goes to its close affinity and thus joining with it, goes to the lungs, and having reached the lungs, the carbon dioxide, if it be carbon dioxide, is expelled; then the sodium goes back to the sodium chloride again. Thus we see, the loose affinity merely keeps these policemen of the system ready to escort carbon dioxide out of the system, and what applies to carbon dioxide here, applies to the other poisonous gases of the system in other ways.

Sodium in the organic form is, therefore, the means of eliminating from the system poisonous gases and acids, but when it becomes inorganic, bound in close affinity, it does not exercise this function. It follows, therefore, that in order to get this efferent principle it is

necessary that the salts be organic, bound together in loose affinity.
The mineral salt is always inorganic; the vegetable salt organic when
not cooked. The giving of mineral drugs is consequently improper; they
will not have this efferent action; this can be secured only by the use
of vegetables in the uncooked form.

The way to take medicine is, therefore, to eat it in the form of
food, and to eat it raw. These salts are contained in fruits, nuts,
cereals, and a number of vegetables and in herbs more than the vegetable
fruits. There are more of them in spinach than in anything else, though
cabbage, cauliflower and kale contain quite a good deal; also the vegetable fruits, sweet peppers, egg plant, tomatoes, and cucumbers are
found to be quite rich in the efferent salts.

A patient with any of these uric acid diseases should consequently
be put on a diet of green herbs in the form of salads, such as kale,
cauliflower, cabbage, spinach, asparagus, mustard greens, and lettuce.
Celery is also good, and the vegetable fruits such as tomatoes, cucumbers, egg plant, sweet peppers, etc., also the fruits such as apples
and pears will be found very advantageous. Ripe olives when not preserved in salt, are excellent also, because of the large quantity of efferent salts contained in them, particularly potassium. Melons are
one of the greatest storehouses of efferent salts and should be eaten
freely in troubles of this kind. If these herbs and vegetable fruits and
other fruits are eaten in proper quantities it will be found they will
soon supply the organic salts in sufficient quantity to carry out the
uric acid from the system, but it should be borne in mind that all they
can do is to carry this acid to the organs whose duty it is to eliminate
it. They will carry a part of it out through the skin, it is true, but
principally through the kidneys; they will pour it into the kidneys,
as it were. The kidneys must be strengthened in order that they may
eliminate the poisonous acids. It is for this reason that mere dieting
will not cure a disease of this type. It is necessary to resort to
something else. The kidneys must be strengthened and to do this we must
resort to metaphysical treatment. Suggestion is a very good thing —
exercises a great influence. We suggest that the kidneys are working;
the force of them is strengthened and they are eliminating, throwing
out the uric acid, because the kidneys will do what we suggest for them
to do. The kidneys of the patient will obey the physician's suggestion
and do that work; also they will get strength if the suggestion that
they are strong be given, because strength will be imparted to them by
reason of this suggestion.

Likewise, if we resort to the use of magnetism or psychical force
we can do even greater good, because as this is imparted to the kidneys,
or the nerve centers controlling them, they will gain strength and thus
throw out the poison. It is, therefore, necessary in giving a magnetic
treatment, to visualize upon the kidneys, to send the current of mag-

netism there and see them eliminating the poisons; make a picture of
them gathering the uric acid out of the blood, separating it and throwing it into the bladder so that it can be eliminated in the form of urine.
In this way we will be able to remove the poison, and rheumatism, eczema,
scrofula and those diseases will be cured; of course, not overcome because eczema and scrofula are skin diseases due to the elimination of
uric acid through the skin, and so when we have taken out all of the uric
acid from the blood the skin will still be inflamed; the poison will
still be there. In this case it will be found necessary to entirely
magnetize the body and then cause a current of magnetic force to flow
outward through the pores of the skin, dissolving the poison that is there
in the skin and taking it out in the form of an ether, and you have got
to see it, to see this magnetic force flowing outward, the healthy aura
carrying out the aura of the disease until it is entirely eliminated.
Likewise, you have got to treat the joints, or the muscles in a case of
rheumatism, causing the healthy ether to flow through and to drive out
the ether of the disease, and carry it out of the system completely because it permeates the entire system, and you may heal the body but if
this condition is in the etheric double, if you do not throw off the
etheric counterpart of the uric acid, you will find it will poison the
system again; will descend and accumulate in the system and the patient
will have to be cured over and over again.

As we thus accomplish the work of freeing the system from uric
acid, we cure those diseases; but Bright's Disease, being a disease of
the kidney itself, presents greater difficulties. In this case we must
treat the organ by sending a current of magnetism through it and rebuilding the tissue that has been taken away, that has been consumed.
This must be built, and as it is rebuilt, replaced, the kidney is built
up, becomes firm and solid and is able to do its work properly. Then it
will be found, to be relieved of this specific condition, it must receive more vitality so that it can throw off the uric acid.

Now, what is it that causes the perishing of the kidney? It is the
accumulation of the acid there faster than the kidney can get rid of
it which causes the poisoning of the tissue; therefore, the treatment
must be to give strength to the kidney and to stimulate its throwing off
tendency so that it will be helped to eliminate and get rid of this
poison more and more, faster and faster, and as it gets rid of it, is
cleaned off, then we must build up the tissue by the action of magnetism,
by the use of mental picturing and by the activity of the creative energy
as it is sent there. Suggestion should be used to this end, also and by
building up the kidney in this way and by helping it to get rid of the
uric acid, you will be able to cure Bright's Disease or any of the other
diseases.

To recapitulate briefly, the treatment for all uric acid diseases
must be:

First — Abstinence from all cooked protein in the diet, and from all protein of any kind for a short time.

Second — A diet largely composed of vegetables and vegetable fruits, eaten raw, supplemented by other fruits and nuts containing efferent salts, but preferably fruits and nuts, owing to the large quantity of protein in the latter.

Third — Suggestion as a means of stimulating the activity of the kidneys.

Fourth — The use of magnetism to help the kidneys to throw off the poison.

Fifth — Certain exercises, Yoga practices, that will be found advantageous in stimulating the kidneys and other excretal organs.

Sixth — The practice of concentrating on the patient, causing a healthy ether to permeate his etheric double and driving outward the diseased ether until it is driven through the pores of the skin and thus escapes from the patient.

Seventh — For Bright's Disease, the treatment of the kidney itself in order that it may be built up and nourished — the replenishing of the perishing tissue.

If all these factors are intelligently combined, it will be found that all Uric Acid Diseases, Bright's Disease included, when not progressed too far, can be cured without fail; but it is utterly useless to try to cure them without regulating the diet of the patient, because he is continually putting into the system the very same poison which is causing the disease.

Bear in mind that Uric Acid Diseases are merely the manifestations of poison which is in the system, the outward manifestation a curative attempt in other words, and the disease, therefore, can be properly cured only by getting rid of the uric acid, and this cannot be done while the patient is continually accumulating more and more of it; but free the system from Uric Acid and every Uric Acid Disease will disappear in a comparatively short time.

LESSON ON

STARCH POISON

One of the greatest sources of disease is the poison which accumulates in the system from eating too much cooked starch. The starch globule is by nature provided with a woody envelope which entirely covers it, excluding the saliva, so that it is with considerable difficulty it is digested. It is not true, however, that the saliva is absolutely unable to act upon this woody envelope. That is the theory ordinarily held by physicians, but it is inaccurate. The saliva can act upon this and dissolve it and thus get to the starch globule so as to act upon it, but it requires a considerable quantity of saliva to accomplish this feat. It is with considerable difficulty that this work can be accomplished, therefore, there is but a small quantity of starch that can be digested in this way. As a result, there is no danger of starch poisoning where the starch is taken into the stomach in the raw form. That which is not dissolved and thus acted upon by the saliva will simply pass through the system without any change taking place, will go through the bowels and escape; but when cooking takes place, when fire is applied to the starch, this woody envelope is dissolved by the heat. The result is, the saliva comes directly in contact with the starch and thus transmutes it. It should be understood, also, that the starch is no longer organic; that is, the molecules bound together in loose affinity, but by the action of heat, has become inorganic, this loose affinity having been broken up and they are now bound together in close affinity or else not connected at all. When the starch is taken into the mouth in this form the saliva transmutes it, not into grape sugar, as it would if it were in the raw state, but into Glucose, and in this shape it enters the chyle and thus passes into the blood. The same thing takes place that takes place when you put cooked starch in water, that thick, milky solution is formed, and thus it mixes with the blood. If you were to put raw starch into the system that way, it would not mix at all, and unless it were changed into the chyle proper and could become a part of the

41

constituency of the blood, it would simply pass away without any mixture at all; but when cooked, it produces this condition in the blood; the blood becomes poisoned by it and in time it acts upon the tissues so that they become permeated with this glucose. The system undertakes to eliminate the glucose; the blood wants to get rid of it; it tries to purify itself by eliminating the glucose. It does this by transferring it to the tissue and a number of diseases grow up out of this effort of nature to eliminate the glucose from the blood. The mucous membrane receives the glucose and undertakes to get rid of it, and a cold is nothing in the world but the condition of the mucous membrane growing out of this glucose poisoning. The glucose is carried to the mucous membrane and there is being discharged, and a cold is, consequently the effort of Nature to eliminate the glucose from the mucous membrane. A change of air does not originate a cold, it simply precipitates one; the origin of the cold is in the glucose that is poisoning the tissue. A change in the temperature or a change in the state of humidity in the atmosphere, exposure, anything of that kind, simply precipitates this poisonous influence that is operative in the system, causing it to come to the surface and is, therefore, a healing action. It is a curative act on the part of nature – is a form of elimination.

When there is so much glucose in the system that it cannot be gotten rid of in this way, but continues to pass through the mucous membrane, becoming chronic and lasting an indefinite period of time, it becomes catarrh. All of these diseases such as Hay Fever, Influenza, Diphtheria and Tonsilitis, are manifestations of the same thing. Not that we would deny the germ of diphtheria, for instance, or affirm that there is no truth in what physicians teach in regard to the nature of those diseases, but this we would affirm and that absolutely without question or limitation; those diseases can operate only in a fruitful soil; they must have congenial environment and that congenial environment or fruitful soil is provided by tissue permeated with glucose and in no other way, consequently, all of those diseases are where there has been an effort on the part of Nature to eliminate; attempts to get rid of the glucose. The disease of bronchitis is another of the same class; lagrippe and everything of that description are simply the efforts of Nature to eliminate this glucose. Lupus is another one of the same class, a disease where the system is eliminating glucose, through the skin and so much of it is brought to the surface that in time it starts up tuberculosis of the skin, and then the germs can get in their work.

Now, those remedies are only valuable as corrective for lupus that help to eliminate the poison from the skin, such as the Violet ray, the Finsen light, the Sun baths – anything of that kind or other treatments which have the influence of inducing copious perspiration and stimulating the eliminating action of the skin. Whenever you do this and get rid of the glucose, the disease will disappear.

Consumption or Pulmonary tuberculosis is another form of the same trouble. It is a case where the glucose has accumulated in the lungs and this provided a favorable feeding ground for the bacilli tuberculosi. Consumption is, therefore, the effect of Starch Poison, just like all the other diseases of this type. If the glucose accumulates in the lungs a case of consumption is inevitable. If it can be kept out, there is no danger.

The treatment for consumption must, therefore, first of all, be the elimination of all forms of cooked starch from the diet because it was in this way that so much starch accumulated in the system, more than the nutrition could make use of. We must confine the patient to a diet of raw starch. What is it that must be eliminated then? Potatoes of every kind, because they are almost exclusively starch; also carrots and parsnips and every thing of that kind, if cooked; cooked chestnuts, because they contain quite a quantity of starch. That crowning iniquity of modern degeneration, cooked bananas, must also be eliminated for they are almost entirely formed of starch; white bread of every description, in fact all kinds of cooked bread excepting gluten bread, where the starch has been taken out of the wheat — that may be used — but all other forms of bread, all cooked cereals, legumens, unless eaten while green, and everything of that description must be eliminated from the diet. Let the diet consist of nuts and fruits, mainly. Sugar and protein, with fats also should be a considerable part of the diet. It is best to entirely eliminate starch for a few days and then begin on a diet of raw starch with the other foods. Do not follow the theory, however, that a meat diet is necessary in cases of consumption. There is no truth in this, but what is important is a diet of protein, mainly. Sugar is not a good substitute for starch because they are both carbon-hydrates and are very closely allied. The other elements are fats and protein and should be employed freely.

The use of meat has grown out of the idea that it was the only form or at least, the best form in which protein could be made use of. It has also been supposed to be the best form of fat. Cod liver oil and all those abominations are not at all necessary, but a diet of nuts, nut butter and olive oil, — vegetable fats are what are required.

A great many physicians think that animal food is necessary for the consumptive. This is not true, either. There is no occasion for the use of animal food at all. Eggs, butter and milk are not needed at all and a diet of nuts and acid fruits, with plenty of fats as contained in vegetable oils will be found to give much better results than any form of animal food.

The patient suffering from any of these troubles should be in the open air, as much as possible; as the oxygen he gets in the system will have the effect of building up the fires of the body and driving out and destroying this accumulated glucose. Thus the health will be greatly improved. Also, the Prana which the patient will get in the air and from the sunshine will help to build him up and strengthen his system and enable him to throw off those poisons.

It should be borne in mind that the perspiration which one throws off by reason of physical exercise has the influence of carrying away the poisonous glucose and in this way, Turkish baths will be found advisable, but should not be taken to excess, in which case there will be danger of the system being weakened and depleted of its vitality.

Another thing that should be borne in mind is that all those types of disease are due to a magnetic condition of the Electro-Magnetic forces of the body; that is to say, the accumulation of glucose in the system produces this magnetic condition, and the equilibrium is overturned, the system gets weak in the electrical force, and a cure can be brought about only by restoring the equilibrium, consequently it will be found advantageous to increase the electrical force in the body. Any kind of treatment which will lead to that result will be found to be advantageous.

The patient, should in addition to the diet above prescribed, eat freely of green herbs and vegetable fruits in the raw state so as to secure as much of the eliminant salts as possible. In this way he will be able to eliminate the principal part of the glucose poison. He should also be given treatment by suggestion and magnetically, for the purpose of dissolving and driving out the glucose from the system, driving it through the tissues and also out of the blood; see it dissolve, throw it into the ether and then cause this ether to flow outward through the pores of the skin until it is entirely eliminated from the system. If you have to treat a case of catarrh this current of magnetic force should be made to permeate the body and gradually be thrown out through the mucous membrane, with a picture of dissolving, throwing off and carrying out all the poison, and also all of the inflammation — everything of that kind. See it sweeping out and cleaning out of the membrane all of this poison, inflammation and everything of that kind. If it be Lupus, then let it go to the surface and in your mind's eye see it dissolving and carrying this poison out through the pores of the skin, allaying the inflammation and cleansing the skin. If it be consumption, you must work on the lungs and dissolve the glucose, throw it into the ether and drive it out through the lungs; destroy the disease germs, dissolve all the corruption or pus that may be in the lungs, and everything of that kind — all the diseased poisonous matter. This must be dissolved into the ether and driven completely out of the body and beyond the Aura. Then, the tissue, if it be decaying or eating away, must be healed up. When all

44

the diseased tissue has been dissolved and carried out, then it must
be treated and healed up and this must also be done by Magnetism;
then, when you have healed it up, if you are treating metaphysically,
you may continue your treatments to make the cells grow back again and
cause the cavities to be filled up with new cellular tissue. Of course,
you have to keep the picture quite distinct and see the cells as such,
growing back, going back into place. If you do not, instead of forming
new cells you will simply form a mass of connective tissue, which will
be better than the cavity, but nothing like so desirable as to have
the cavity filled up with new cells and air passages; but you can
completely restore the lung by treatment of this kind.

By the combination of proper dieting, proper exercises and fresh
air, sunlight, etc., hygienic methods of living, with suggestive
therapeutics and magnetic healing — or the higher forms of healing are
still better — it is possible to cure any case of consumption where
the patient has lungs enough to enable him to live until you have time
to accomplish the cure. There is no question about your ability to
restore the lungs if your patient lives long enough for you to do it.
The only danger is that he will die before you have time to get in the
work. But with the method herein outlined, it is possible to cure any
case of consumption in the world.

Fresh air, sunshine, plenty of exercise, the electrical principle in place of the magnetic, and the proper diet as herein
directed, coupled with the proper mental attitude, and plenty of
magnetism (but the magnetism should be positive, that is to say electrical force rather than negative or magnetic) will cure any case of
consumption in the world, where the patient has strength enough to
hold out until the treatment has time to get in its work on his organism.

Remember, the bacilli tuberculosi operate only in congenial
soil. They are not the cause of consumption, but rather the effect,
the instrument of destroying the poison which has accumulated in the
system and, therefore, an effort on the part of nature toward a cure.
They are the efforts of nature to get rid of the poison that you have
placed in the body. Usually they kill the body in clearing out the
glucose, but the proper treatment and diet will relieve the disease of
so much rubbish and will, therefore, make it quite easy for the glucose
to be eliminated and permit the patient to live.

It should be borne in mind that cooked starch, when taken into
the system goes through a process of fermentation and all of the grape
sugar or glucose, rather, which goes through this fermentative process
is transmuted into alcohol, excepting that which goes into the formation of carbonic acid gas. The poisoning resulting to the system from
carbonic acid gas, is, therefore, due largely to the fermentation of
the starch or rather the glucose that comes from grape sugar. The
dangers coming from carbonic acid gas or from carbon dioxide are

largely due to the practice of eating cooked starch. An avoidance of a diet of cooked starch will greatly relieve the system from the poison of carbonic acid gas.

L E S S O N   O N

S U G A R   P O I S O N

The type of disease which we will consider this time is that which might be denominated "Sugar Poison," that is to say, those diseases which are the efforts of nature to eliminate the surplus cooked sugar which is accumulated in the system.

The longer we study the food problem, the more clearly it will be impressed upon our minds, that raw food will never accumulate in the system.

The stomach and other digestive organs can digest only a sufficient quantity to satisfy the demands of nutrition when in the raw state, but when in the cooked state it becomes so much easier to digest that the stomach and other organs will digest the food and thus a larger quantity is converted into chyle and enters the blood in that state, much more than the system really requires and consequently, it cannot be made into sound tissue, but accumulates in the system in this form and then in the course of time must be eliminated in some way. The system then in its effort to eliminate this poison will produce certain diseased conditions.

Now, there is one point which you must clearly understand namely, disease is NOT an evil. Disease is an effort on the part of nature to eliminate poison. It is an effort to cure and consequently is desirable compared to that state of poison which it attempts to eliminate.

Now, when we know this fact we can understand the desirability of giving to the system only a sufficient quantity of food to supply nutrition; but when the food is cooked, all that enters the stomach goes through the digestive processes; therefore, the only safe course is to eat only uncooked food and in this way the system cannot be overfed; it will simply pass out through the alimentary canal.

When sugar is cooked there is a chemical change which takes place, the result being that it goes through a process of fermentation when it enters the stomach and by this process of fermentation, a large quantity of it is converted into alcohol; in fact, all of it which is digested by the process of fermentation. The balance goes through a change which converts it into carbonic acid gas. Now, that part which is not fermented is taken into the system in the form of organic sugar and then is used by the system in that way, but it is much more difficult to organize this cooked sugar into tissue than to organize the uncooked sugar. As a result the gas, of course, poisons the system and must in the course of time be eliminated; but also the sugar enters the system, and that which has been converted into alcohol has precisely the same effect on the system as any other alcohol will have.

Now, it may not seem reasonable, but let us say absolutely that there are people, to our personal knowledge, who never touch alcoholic liquor, who are tetotalers, and yet they have the red nose and, in fact, every sympton of alcoholism, and those persons will be found to be heavy eaters of cooked sugar. We once knew one, who at every meal, would take sugar, make a syrup, and eat a teacupful of the sugar-syrup. The way he did it, — he would set it down by his plate and whenever he got ready to eat a morsel of bread he would dip the slice of bread into the syrup and then eat it — saturated with syrup. All the bread he used he ate that way; in fact, he always ate a teacupful of sugar-syrup besides sweetening everything he ate. He would take a tumbler and would put in all the sugar that would dissolve in a tumbler of hot water. It showed itself in his life, in his body and even in his mind. He acted like a drunken man, although he never touched alcohol.

This evil is avoided by the eating of sugar in the raw state; it is not organic, but inorganic sugar, which ferments and makes alcohol. By cooking sugar it is disorganized and thus easily goes through this process of fermentation. If you want to avoid this alcoholic effect, the only way is to take organic, that is to say, raw sugar into the system.

Now, when we take a certain quantity of cooked sugar into the system it not only produces this alcoholic, but carbonic acid poison as well, and it also enters in the form of inorganic sugar into the system, saturating the tissue and producing the poisonous effect. In this state man would not live so very long if it were not for the action of the kidneys in eliminating this poison from the system. Now, as long as the kidneys are able to keep out a sufficient quantity of it and eliminate it, there will be no serious results; but sometimes the kidneys become overworked and are unable to handle this surplus quantity of cooked sugar. They cannot get it out of the system, or in doing so, have become overworked and become deranged. Diabetes is nothing but the result of cooked sugar in the system. No case of chronic diabetes has ever been cured by the ordinary medical practice, and diabetes in the chronic form cannot be cured permanently without a change in the diet. If you will eliminate cooked sugar from the diet, you will have removed the cause of diabetes. That does not mean that the patient will get well immediately because when it manifests in the form of chronic diabetes there has usually been an accumulation of ten or twelve years of sugar poison and it is necessary that we get rid of that poison before we can ever hope to cure the patient.

What then are we going to do? Well, we must first eliminate cooked sugar from the diet so that there is no more put into the system. Then we must adopt a diet which will help to eliminate this sugar and then we must give such treatment, metaphysical treatment we mean, as will tend to help the elimination, to get rid of this poison. At the same time the kidneys must be strengthened because they are eliminating this poison from the blood and they must be strengthened so as to do more work. At the same time if there be any organic defect it must be built up and cured.

In the first place, let us consider the elimination of cooked sugar. What foods must we eliminate in order to get rid of cooked sugar? In the first place, we must eliminate all commercial sugar because it is all cooked, whether cane, maple or beet sugar. It must all be entirely eliminated from the diet, consequently we must have nothing to do with it at all. We must eliminate pies, cakes and everything that is sweet which has been cooked. Preserves and canned fruit, in fact all of cooked food of every description must be eliminated, also evaporated fruit, and every kind of fruit, in fact, which has gone through the process of cooking. Candy must be eliminated; the person must not be permitted to eat anything of that kind, anything of a sweet character which has gone through the process of cooking. Boiled milk which, with so many people, is such a great palliative of all the ills to which flesh is heir, must be eliminated because it has poisoned the sugar contained in the milk, being in the cooked state.

You say then where are you going to get the sugar required for nutrition? You must use organic sugar; that means use fruits in the natural state, either sun-dried or else fresh. You must use those fruits; you may use honey also, as it is not a cooked sugar, although it is not so desirable as the natural fruit sugar contained in sweet fruits. Ripe bananas in the raw state are very desirable, excellent food, but should never be cooked. That crowning abomination of desolation, that has entered into the dietary of modern life — fried bananas, must certainly be eliminated in every case of this kind. St. John's bread is an excellent form of raw sugar.

Now, no matter how much you eat in that state it will not hurt you for the simple reason it may give you a case of diarrhea, but you will soon get over it.

Of all the ridiculous nonsense in the world one of the greatest is the idea that it will not do for children to eat raw fruit. People are afraid it will make them sick to eat fruit in a raw state, but will let them sit at the table and stuff themselves on evaporated fruits, preserves, jellies and all kinds of cooked fruit, the only form in which it can hurt them, because it gets into the system, otherwise it simply passes through the alimentary canal. We find this kind of dietary regime will cut off all sugar poison. Syrups of all kinds must also be eliminated.

How are we going to get rid of that sugar which has already accumulated in the system? In the same way we get rid of all the other food poisons, namely, by taking into the system large quantities of the efferent salts, sodium, potassium, calcium, magnesium, phosphorus and silicon, and these efferent salts will help to carry out of the system those poisons, no matter what they may be. They will carry them out through the lungs and thus the blood will be purified from that condition and those poisons will be carried out of the blood. Now, this is a natural way of purifying the blood, by the different salts carrying impurities out of the blood through the lungs and throwing it out.

The way, as we have said before, to secure the salts is by eating green vegetables such as spinach, cabbage, cauliflower, lettuce and other vegetables along those lines; also it may be secured in large quantities from the vegetable fruits, — cucumbers, tomatoes, sweet peppers, egg plant, and from melons of all descriptions; also from squash, pumpkin and such. Among the fruits the richest in the salts is undoubtedly the olive, that is ripe olives, dried not pickled olives. Olives that are soaked in brine are of no value, and, in fact, are detrimental, the same as everything else that has been pickled; also practically all nuts contain considerable quantities of those salts.

Among tree fruits, the apple, the fig, and the date contain considerable quantities.

By eating these foods you get the salts into the system so that those poisons are eliminated in this way.

Now, by adopting a diet of this kind, by drinking considerable water and by bathing so as to help the system throw off those poisons, you accomplish all that can be done by naturepathic treatment.

Here we have to introduce the metaphysical treatment. Remember that for all this type of diseases such as diabetes and everything of that type which is caused by sugar poison, the treatment is practically the same. Of course, if it effects different organs, those organs must be strengthened, but in a general way, the treatment is the same. For this reason we must deal with them collectively.

Remember the thing you want to accomplish is the elimination of this poison from the blood and tissue, so if you are giving treatment by suggestion, offer your suggestions in this way for this purpose; direct them to the destruction or disintegration, disorganization, dissolution of this sugar poison which is in the blood, so that it may be dissolved, and then by this process throw it into the ether and have it flow out through the system. If you are practicing suggestive therapeutics, you want suggestion of that kind, also you want to suggest that the sugar poison which has accumulated in the tissue, is disintegrating, is dissolving, throwing it into the ether, and let it pass out from the system. Also, stimulate the kidneys, having the poison go to the kidney and pass out through them as the sewerage system for this purpose, and strengthen them. If there be any weakness there, send a current of vitality to the kidneys that they may be able to perform their work properly.

If you are giving treatment by magnetism, treat the same way, only send a current of magnetism through and through the body of your patient, not to any particular locality, but let it go from the crown of the head to the sole of the feet, permeating every tissue, and cell of his being, and as it goes through thus, you want, by a process of mental picturing, to dissolve this poison; this inorganic sugar must be dissolved, disintegrated and thrown into the ether, and then as you continue to send more and more of this magnetic force through the body, drive this poison out of the system, out of the surface, and let it flow out until it comes to the pores of the skin and outside of the body a considerable distance. Let this Aura stream forth, and this Aura must be magnetism which you are pouring in.

The same is true in treating by spiritual, psychical, or Divine Healing. It is the same process, dissolving the poison, throwing it into the ether and then letting it flow out through the tissue and through the pores of the skin until it has been expelled from the body.

At the same time you want to act upon the blood; magnetize the blood, throwing a powerful charge of this current through it. The blood becomes magnetic.

In this state you want to dissolve the sugar poison, disintegrate, throw it into the ether and drive out and even burn it up. Imagine a fire raging through and through the blood and the system, which is burning up and consuming all these poisons until they have entirely gone and the system is cleared up.

Now, remember in all those methods of treatment you do not want to take the attitude that it is going to do this by and by, but always you must maintain the attitude that this is now taking place. You see it is doing this, it is taking place, see it with your mind's eye, watch the process going on just as you want it to go on. Never for one moment tolerate the idea that it is going to do it by and by, but see it doing it now, and as you make your suggestions, make them in that way — that it is doing it now, and always at the end, see the system entirely cleared of everything of the kind so that the sugar poison is entirely eliminated from the body.

By processes of treatment of this kind you will be able to reach the most perfect results, but in no other way is it possible to cure diseases of this character.

By combining the Naturepathic and Metaphysical treatments in this way we will be able to eliminate the poisons and thus the disease itself will cease because its cause will have been removed; we will have taken away the poison which expressed itself in the form of disease; there will be nothing there to cause the disease any longer, consequently, it disappears by itself, but in no other way is it possible to cure a disease of this kind.

It is, therefore, utterly useless to attempt to cure a patient unless you can induce him to quit eating cooked sugar. You may by powerful force which you may bring to bear, eliminate all the poison in the system or destroy it so that its action is neutralized, so that the body is clear of poison. In that case your patient will be well, but remember if he goes on eating cooked sugar; in the course of time his body will again be filled with the poison and the same disease will come back and that is why the work of healers is found to be not permanent, the same as that of physicians, because they do not stop the cause, and it reproduces the disease in time.

Also, you may eliminate enough of the poison so that the system will be cleared of it, and it will not manifest itself in the form of that disease again, but in the course of time the poison will increase and the patient will be sick again.

We must, therefore, understand that it is only by the permanent elimination of this poison that it is possible for one to be cured of diseases of this description, therefore, do not let yourself be drawn into the practice of many physicians of curing symptoms, but know that the only way by which it is possible to cure disease is to remove the cause, and the only cause of all this type is the accumulation in the system of the poison coming from cooked sugar.

LESSON ON

CANCER

CANCER is caused by the waste from meat; not by protein or anything of that kind, but by the waste which is left from meat. Now the
reason why this is so, is because the waste left by meat is in
particles larger and also traveling in a larger circuit in their revolution than the affinity of the kidney can eliminate. They have a
larger circuit and consequently the kidneys are unable to eliminate
that waste.

Now, the kidneys are provided by nature for the purpose of
eliminating waste from the particular organism that possesses those
kidneys. An animal kidney will eliminate animal waste, but a human
kidney can eliminate only the human waste — the waste that accumulates
through the activities of the human body. Now, unfortunately for meat
eating people, their kidneys are not adapted to the elimination of
animal waste. The vessels are not large enough, consequently the animal
waste cannot pass through the kidney and thus be transferred to the
urine, consequently it cannot be eliminated, but remains in the system.

The chemical food value of meat is not taken into consideration
here. Cooked protein does not cause cancer; no kind of cooked food
has such influence; it is solely the animal waste and because the animal waste cannot be eliminated through the kidneys, it remains in the
blood and in the tissue. We know this is the cause of it, for a number
of reasons.

In the first place, there has never been known a case of cancer
in a nation of vegetarians.

Second: there has never been a case of cancer in a family of
vegetarians who lived in a country where other people were meat eaters.

In the Third place: an individual who was himself a vegetarian
has never been known to have cancer, and lastly, the proper diet will
cure cancer, or at least make it much better.

Now, inasmuch as the waste from meat eating is the cause of cancer, you can readily see that cancer cannot be cured by any method as long as people continue to eat meat. It may be that the individual cancer can be cured, but that waste is still in the system and must manifest itself in some way until we get it out.

Cancer is an effort on the part of Nature to cure this trouble, to eliminate this poison. As it cannot be eliminated through the kidneys, neither can it be eliminated through the bowels, it must get out in some other way; the only way by which this meat waste can escape is in the form of cancer. If there is an abrasion on the surface of the body anywhere it will strongly tend to cause cancer to form there. If there is nothing of the kind, it may form anywhere. It may form on the surface of the body, or it may form on some internal organ, but in every case the formation of the cancer is an effort on the part of the system to eliminate the waste that came from meat.

When the cancer is first formed it appears to have at its base, roots running in, looking like veins, only they are darker, or black, in fact, and running in. These roots which appear, are the streams, so to speak of this waste; that is, it is going forward from different directions and converging in the mass of the cancer. As long as the cancer continues, however, it enlarges and it does so because as it stays there, this meat waste is continually coming to the front; it is continually drawing to that point and, therefore, the increasing size of the cancer simply means that the waste is being taken from the system. In this respect, it is an advantage, and the eating of a cancer is always an advantage to the system unless it goes on to the point where it becomes so large and eats so deeply that it destroys some physical organ or something of the kind. However, of course, it greatly lowers the vitality as the vital energy is necessary to sustain life and sustain the ravages of the cancer, and as it continues to increase and destroy the tissue because of this poison accumulating, as the tissue is being destroyed, it is, therefore, making the building of new tissue more and more necessary as we go on.

Well then, what are we to conclude? We see that the presence of a cancer indicates a continual separating force, an eating, a destruction of the tissue, simply because the meat waste is destructive. This poison is such that it will destroy living tissue; it is a putrifying force and will destroy in the same way that putrid flesh attached to a living body in time act so as to destroy the living tissue. It, therefore, becomes a destructive, eating sore; but we must bear in mind that this is the organization of the waste when allowed to manifest itself. It is not allowed to accumulate and manifest ordinarily, but the poison is still in the system.

Now, a number of diseases are the efforts of Nature to eliminate poison, and in those efforts the body may be so weakened that life will be extinguished. The body may be destroyed, in Nature's efforts to heal. Cancer is an effort to eliminate meat waste, remember, consequently no permanent cure can be accomplished that does not take cognizance of this fact and act accordingly. If we leave the meat waste in the system and continue to feed it by feeding upon meat, we may cure the cancer, but we leave the cause in the system and the next time it may appear on a vital organ, so that life will be extinguished much quicker than it would if the cancer were on the surface of the body.

Many methods have been devised to treat cancer locally. The old idea was to remove it by an operation. This, it is true, will remove the principal part of the cancer, but remember, this is simply a gathering of the cancerous influence. The small veins back of it still remain and they will simply get larger.

To remove a cancer by operation is like removing or filling up a hole filled with water and allowing the stream to keep running in all the time.

The next method which was adapted was the X-Ray, which treats cancer by battering it with the anode and the cathode so that the tissues dissolve; that is better than using the knife, because we can go much farther up and get the roots out to a much greater degree; but still this is simply treating the effect; the cause is left untouched. The Violet Ray and the use of Radium are still better because they dissolve it without the bad effects of the X-Ray, that is, they do not leave a hole, but actually dissolve it; but still those methods are all merely local, merely treatments of an effect, leaving the cause intact.

The use of drugs for cancer is the same way. They may cure the cancer, but leave the cancerous poison in the system.

The only way to permanently cure cancer is by treating this cancerous poison, therefore, the rational treatment of cancer is to first cease eating meat. As long as the patient lives upon a meat diet he can never be cured of cancer; therefore, the first step is to put him on an absolutely vegetarian diet, or, at least a meatless diet. Understand, the use of cheese, butter, milk, eggs, etc., are not detrimental to cancerous treatment; it is meat that must not be used. Put the patient on a meatless diet so that no more of this waste will accumulate in the system. But that is not sufficient to cure. To stop the patient from accumulating any more meat waste is not going to get rid of what has already formed. You must get rid of this in some way, and this can be very greatly aided by proper dieting. What we want to do is to get as much of the efferent salts into the system as possible. The efferent salts are sodium, potassium, calcium, magnesium, silicon and phosphorus. You want to get as much of these salts into the system as possible, because they will combine with the waste and help to eliminate it, and they will also carry this waste to the cancer, and thus, by increasing the cancerous discharge, help to get rid of the waste very quickly.

The foods which contain these salts to a large degree are the herbs, in fact, green vegetables of every description, and spinach, cabbage, cauliflower and kale contain more, perhaps, than any others; also there is a good deal in celery. Among the vegetable fruits also, you will find tomatoes, sweet peppers, egg plant, cucumbers and such contain those salts. Melons and pumpkins contain considerable, and among fruits the apple and the olive. Nuts of all kinds contain a large percentage of those salts.

Now, remember this: these foods contain those salts in the organic form when RAW. Whenever any of them are cooked this salt is disorganized, becomes inorganic and from that time it is unable to perform this function of eliminating the poison from the system. It is no longer a living force, but becomes a chemical deposit in the system.

Organic salt, therefore, does not injure the system, does not lead to old age, etc., but inorganic salt always does. So the vegetables, fruits, etc., must be used in the raw state by every one who would attain the best results along those lines.

One other point you must bear in mind is that the pickling of foods destroys these salts, destroys the form of organization, tears it to pieces, and thus its effectiveness is removed.

Now, when you begin to give a diet of this kind to your patient, you will find the cancer will get much worse, get larger, it will break and begin to run, it will seem to get into a terrible state. This is just what you want to take place. It gets that way simply because there is three or four times the usual quantity of meat waste that has been discharged there, consequently it breaks and runs. When it sloughs off that way, you are getting rid of that waste.

Do not get the idea so many people do, that these foods are not good for cancer, or make the cancer worse. That is the way we cure cancer, by discharging the poison.

However, the cancer may be so far advanced that this kind of treatment will not save the life of the patient. It is quite often the case that you must get rid of the poison in some other way, to keep it from destroying the life of the patient, but this is the way in which cancer must be cured, by ELIMINATING THE MEAT WASTE from the system.

Now, at the time you are treating your patient by this method of diet, you should also employ metaphysical methods of healing to work in conjunction with the treatment. By working in conjunction with it, we mean apply it in such a way as to do the same work as this dietary regime is, namely, carry the meat waste out of the system.

In the first place, you may employ suggestion along this line, for the carrying out of that meat waste, and carrying it out through the cancer, making that the avenue. Make suggestions so as to cause the mind of the patient to bring out this meat waste, bring it to the surface there and eliminate it.

Also in giving Healing Treatments, either Magnetic or any of the higher forms, when you have permeated the patient with the magnetism, the proper thing to do is to bring a current of magnetism through the body and out through this cancer, at the same time picturing the meat waste being separated from the system and in a soluble state, so to speak, in this magnetic force which you have caused to permeate the body of your patient. Draw it out to the surface and carry it out. Let this current of magnetic force flowing from the body, stream out through the cancer, carrying away this waste product.

Also, while treating your patient, you must in this magnetic way disorganize these particles of meat waste; break them up into smaller fragments or better still, dissolve them into the ether, so that instead of being solid matter, they become etheric. Now, in this etheric state, cause this waste to flow out through the tissue, which will be quite easy. Then with your magnetism, make it flow out through the surface, out through the cancer until it has left the body.

Also, you can drive it out through the pores of the skin through the entire being and with each treatment cause it to be driven out this way, through this cancerous opening, so that it will entirely disappear and be dissipated from the system. Next, remember, that by breaking it up into small fragments you make it possible for the kidneys to eliminate the poison which they could not do before, and as the poison is driven out through the cancer in this etheric form, there is, in consequence, much less to be eliminated by the kidneys.

Also, do not lose sight of the fact that you must get the cancerous ether out of the etheric double as well as getting the solid waste out of the gross body.

Next, bear in mind that you must not neglect the local treatment of the cancer as well as the system, and, by the local treatment, we mean that this cancerous tissue which is eating away and poisoning the sound tissue, must also be permeated with magnetism. This tendency must be killed and it must be dissolved into an ether and thrown from the system. It must be entirely removed and pass out, so that it gradually dissolves and passes out into the Aura around the body.

You must kill this cancerous state and remove this tissue in this magnetic way, or by suggestion or by any method of that kind, at the same time you are eliminating it from the system. Do not wait until you have all the waste out of the system before you commence on the cancer. If you do, it may have gone too far, may have destroyed some vital part of the body. Treat them together, but whatsoever you do, do not try to heal up the cancer. Simply eliminate the meat waste from the system and also this cancerous tissue. Concentrate a strong current of vitality so as to intensely vitalize that part of the body, at the same time giving the food which will help to throw off this cancerous poison.

Now remember, if a cancer is on an internal organ you have to use the same method of treatment as you would otherwise, only, of course, you have to visualize upon the organ so that in your mind's eye you can see the cancer. Concentrate your attention and then disorganize the cancer by dissolving the ether and dissolving the cancer itself and throwing it into the form of an ether and letting it saturate the system, so it is broken up, disorganized; then cause this ether to flow out, eliminating it from the system. Make it pass out through the pores of the skin, through the entire body, until it leaves. You must eliminate the poison from the system as you would in the ordinary case of poison, but first you must cause the cancer to disorganize and throw its force out through the system. You must also be sure to build up the tissue of this vital organ. You must vitalize it to a much higher degree than it would otherwise be so as to prevent any disorganizing effect and any eating action of the organ itself.

It is in this way, and in this way only, that internal cancer can be cured.

Now, notice the most effective methods for cancer have been, — speaking of the physical, — the use of the X-Ray, the Violet Ray and Radium, — in other words, the application of electro-magnetic force for the purpose of disorganizing the diseased tissue. That is found to be the most effective method of treatment known to the medical profession. By the use of magnetism we are really employing that in a much higher sense than the physician is able to do. We are concentrating the same force on a higher plane — vital magnetism — to break up and dissolve this diseased tissue and eliminate it from the system.

If you are treating a case of surface cancer, it may be found advisable to place the left — the magnetic hand — that is to say if a man be practicing healing, the right if a woman be practicing — but place the negative hand over the cancer and then in your treatments, while you are driving out the poisonous forces, with the negative hand draw them out, and be very careful in doing this. If you make the slightest slip you are liable to take the cancer yourself, because you are really drawing those forces out into your negative hand, therefore, after you have given a treatment, be sure to concentrate your force very positively and make it flow out. In other words, make this the positive hand for a few minutes; then shake it with all the force you have, as you would shake water off the ends of your fingers, shaking it fifty or a hundred times, vigorously, at the same time, concentrating, visualizing upon a current of magnetism running out through the ends of your fingers. Be careful to be very positive while you are doing this, without questioning your ability to eliminate this poisonous ether; otherwise you will be almost sure to contract a case of cancer.

Also, while treating a patient for cancer do not let any one else stay in the room; there is danger of giving it to others; also it is best not to treat another patient for fifteen or twenty minutes after treating a cancerous patient because there is danger of the evil magnetism effecting the next patient, and the room should be fumigated with incense of a very powerful character, immediately after a treatment of that kind, so as to destroy the poison which is driven out of the system.

If these methods are followed, any case of cancer in the world can be cured in three months, and generally speaking, if not too far gone, a month is sufficient to accomplish a cure, but no method will accomplish permanent results unless the person forever abandons the use of meat. You must bear in mind, however, that abandoning the use of meat does not get rid of the waste already in the system; therefore, you must use methods of the kind described; but by a combination of vegetarianism and a diet of raw food consisting principally of green vegetables, also the employment of suggestion and magnetism in the treatment, in this way, you will accomplish a cure in every instance.

One thing we must call your attention to: Do not follow the practice of placing the positive hand over the cancer and directing the force inward; that method is simply following the methods of operation which are employed by all the physicians. What you want to do is not to drive the force into the cancer, but draw the poison out of the system through the cancer, as the cancer is the effort of Nature to eliminate this waste from meat, and we should co-operate with this effort, work in conjunction with it and by doing this we will be able to hasten the cure.

LESSON ON

OVERFEEDING

One of the greatest causes of disease is Over Eating; — there are quite a number of diseases which grow out of the gorging of the system by over feeding and the consequent accumulation of effete matter in the system. This type is not due to the eating of any kind of food particularly, which is detrimental in itself, but it is more owing to an improper quantity of food than to improper quality.

When we eat, the system takes up as much of the food as it is able to assimilate. This is employed in tissue building and nourishing the system, all that is left from this quantity that is assimilated, remains in the system in the form of waste and must be eliminated in some way, or, if not eliminated, must continue to accumulate.

Diarrhoea, for instance, is nothing in the world but an effort on the part of Nature to eliminate that accumulated waste material from the bowels. The bowels become gorged, as it were, filled with the effete matter and then Nature goes to work to get rid of it; in the ordinary form it cannot be evacuated with sufficient rapidity. The result is, Nature causes the waste material to go through a change which partially decomposes it, throwing it into a watery state which will not be retained by reason of the tenacity of the bowels, and the result is it flows out, and in this watery discharge, eight or ten times as much of the waste material is evacuated from the bowels as would be possible under ordinary circumstances.

Diarrhoea, bear in mind, is not an evil, but it is an effort on the part of Nature to clean out the bowels. Then it should never be checked; there is no more pernicious practice than the effort to check a diarrhoea; if it were not for the diarrhoea, you would die, — it is the effort on the part of Nature to eliminate this accumulated effete matter. Let the diarrhoea alone; quit eating. Go on a Fast just as long as the diarrhoea lasts, because the diarrhoea is caused by the accumulation of too much waste in the system, and you should abstain from food; drink plenty of water to help clean out the system. Do not undertake to stop or suppress any of these out of the ordinary activities of the system, but, on the contrary, co-operate with Nature in accomplishing the purification of the system along this line, and as you co-operate with Nature, you will find that Nature will accomplish her purposes and thus relieve the system from this accumulated waste.

Now, it may be, in certain cases, necessary to regulate, to a certain extent, this evacuation; you may need a means for partially checking it; because there will be so much of this waste substance accumulated in the system and in the bowels that it will take so long to clean it out, and the discharge will be so violent that in certain instances there is danger of ulceration of the bowels. In this case, it is of the greatest importance that we clean out the bowels gradually. We should fast and at the same time, we may check it a little if it is going too far, but not with the effort of suppression.

Flux is another one of the diseases which grow out of this practice of gorging the bowels. Flux is simply a chronic case of diarrhoea. It is so because there has been an accumulation in the bowels and not only there, but throughout the system, and as the bowels are evacuated, the waste material throughout the system is carried back into the bowels and thus this drain is kept up.

Another thing that we must bear in mind, however, is that in case of flux, the system becomes so deranged by reason of the continuous accumulation of effete matter and the necessity of continually dissolving and liquifying this waste, that it may be carried away, that it gets to dissolving pure food in this way also, so that, which is not naturally waste goes through this chemical change and thus is eliminated in the form of waste. In this way the system is robbed of its proper nourishment because it is not simply the waste, but also the proper and natural nourishment which is thrown off in this liquid state and carried away.

While in the case of flux we cannot employ the fasting treatment, because it will take so long to train Nature back into this, its proper channel and way, that we must practice abstinence rather than fasting; that is, we must adopt a diet which will not accumulate, which will give only the proper nourishment. We should also in this case, avoid those foods which will cause fermentation, and that means all kinds of acid foods; we must use only such foods as will go into the building of tissues without any fermentative waste. Next, use those foods which will help to eliminate waste, and those are green herbs, etc.

As we have shown in the previous lessons, we must also use foods which will prevent any irritation. That means that we must not use any salt or animal fat in the food, and we must have everything sufficiently fine. What we mean by fine is, coarse cereals, and anything of that kind which would have a tendency to irritate the bowels, must be avoided.

In order to avoid these diseases, therefore, (flux, we mean, and diarrhoea) we must help nature to eliminate the waste properly, and at the same time not permit the system to throw into this watery state, good, proper nourishment. Be sure to cut down the diet to about the limit which the system can subsist upon. Then give treatments metaphysically for the flux condition; treat the bowels and the system generally; give them strength, pour a flood of vitality in, so that they will be able to perform their functions in the proper manner, without this improper dissolution, so to speak, of the food.

Another disease of the same type which is due to the same cause, and is an aggravated form of diarrhoea, is cholera morbus, and must be treated in the same way. Cholera itself, is due largely to the same condition; not that we deny there being a cholera germ, not that we should say that cholera is not a contageous disease, but we say that the cholera germ can operate only in the system which is poisoned by the accumulation of effete matter. If a person's body is entirely clear of effete matter, it is perfectly safe for him to nurse cholera patients without any fear of taking the contagion. It is only because the bowels become clogged with effete matter; the blood is charged with it; the whole system, the very tissue is permeated with it; it is for this reason and this reason only that cholera is a menace to life and health.

Let us see now, what the treatment for cholera should be. First of all, we must get rid of this accumulated effete matter; that is the first thing to do, therefore, we must keep the bowels open and get rid of this as fast as possible; also place the patient on such a diet as will help him to get rid of the effete matter. Pay no attention to the germs. Purify the system. At the same time, remember that cholera is due to an intensely electrical condition of the system, as we will show in a future lesson. It is an electrical condition of the system which produces cholera, but this loading of the bowels and the system with effete matter is what provides a basis for cholera. It is what enables this electrical condition to manifest. Now, the thing you want to do is, of course, to establish a magnetic condition of the system and this magnetic condition will throw off the accumulated effete matter. So, in treating metaphysically, you want to make the body magnetic rather than electrical; that is to say, if you are a man, you want to treat the person with your left hand, and the man should treat the patient with the left hand because the magnetic force is in the right hemisphere of the brain and goes through the left hand, and — well in fact in either case that is true, the woman the same as the man. The left hand is the magnetic hand. However, magnetic healing treatments given by the woman will be found to be more effective in cases of cholera than when given by a man. Dysentery is also due to the same cause.

Constipation is largely due to the accumulation of effete matter in the system so that the bowels become charged and then being full, they will not admit of the proper activity. The motion of the bowels which helps the elimination, which moves the contents along and helps in the elimination, also the peristaltic action of the bowels is not permitted because of the bowels being fully swollen out so to speak, therefore, constipation is the result, and in curing constipation you have got to get rid of this accumulated waste and prevent its future accumulation. In order to prevent constipation you must have something to help the peristaltic action of the bowels. The best thing for that purpose is green vegetables used in the raw form, as they do not become so packed, and by reason of the slight irritation to the walls of the bowels, will permit the peristaltic action. If you can't get these, or if you do not want to use this method, if you do not want to eat vegetables, then cereals will help this peristaltic action; and cereals for this purpose should be coarsely ground and they should also contain bran as this will greatly assist in the peristaltic elimination. Further, the use of nuts may be found beneficial; if they are used for this purpose, they should never be blanched, but the outer skin should be allowed to remain because of this. Fruit should not be pared, but the parings should be eaten with the fruit, as it will help this same peristaltic action.

The greatest cause of constipation, probably, is the use of white bread. The starch being cooked, is eaten and forms a pasty substance which seals up the bowels. This may be greatly relieved by the use of coarse ground cereal breads, etc. But also, bear in mind that for constipation a great deal of water must be drunk. Under certain conditions, the use of the method of flushing the colon may be found advantageous, but ordinarily we do not recommend it. It is unnatural, and it should be borne in mind that any unnatural method of treatment is, generally speaking, disadvantageous. Liquids should enter the system through the mouth and not otherwise. Consequently, ordinarily speaking, we do not favor it. The drinking of an abundance of water will answer the purpose in a much more natural way as it has to go somewhere — it has to escape. Of course, a great deal will pass through the kidneys, but it is objected that the kidneys are overworked, that the kidneys therefore, will be worked more than normal; that is all right; the work of the kidneys carries away a good deal of waste through the kidneys.

However, in constipation you will give those treatments largely for the effect of loosening the bowels, of removing the resistance, so that they may be evacuated, also to increase the peristaltic action.

One of the diseases also caused by this kind of debauchery is fever. There is not a fever in the world that is not due solely to the accumulation of effete matter in the system; the system cannot get rid of it, it cannot wash it all away, hence there is a lot of effete matter, accumulated in the tissues which we cannot get rid of, the bowels will not eliminate it, it cannot be gotten rid of otherwise; hence what does the system do? Why, it simply builds a fire to burn up the waste just as we, in ordinary life, kindle fires and burn up the waste around the house, when we get so much we cannot get rid of it in any other way. The fever is a fire which nature has kindled for the purpose of burning up this waste material, therefore, a fever is not an evil, but is an effort on the part of nature to accomplish a cure. What, then are we to do? Why, obviously, we should quit eating while the fever lasts; quit filling up the system with effete matter and, of course, if the fever lasts long enough it may be necessary for us to eat a little something, but just enough to sustain life and let the fever go on, let it burn up and consume this waste material. Of course, if it gets too high, then it is better to lower it, to reduce the fever, but let it go ahead until it consumes the waste material.

Typhoid fever never would exist were it not for the fact that the patient is filled up from head to feet with effete matter, is entirely poisoned with it, which this fever has to consume and which would require quite a length of time to consume it. It would take so long to consume this waste material and that is really why it takes so long for a case of typhoid fever.

Now, the old conception of the doctors that typhoid fever must not be broken up, but allowed to run its course, was proven sound; that doctrine is sound; the fever is to be allowed to go on until it has accomplished the burning up of all this effete matter; and the modern method of curing a case of typhoid fever in a few days are wrong. They may do it, that is true, but remember, they have left the poison in the system unless they go to work and get rid of that poison first; then they can cure it.

Now, of course, if they get rid of it, then the very cause of the fever has been removed, the fire goes out for the want of fuel. It is true, however, that we can cure typhoid fever in a short time by metaphysical healing methods. The way we do this is to dissolve this effete matter into an ether and drive it out of the system, so that the work which it would require nature two months, perhaps, to accomplish even by the use of high fevers, is by this method, accomplished in a few days, or, if you have sufficient healing power, in a few hours, or a few minutes. The only need of a fever is to get the effete matter out of the system and if you can dissolve that in the ether and drive the thing entirely out, you could cure the fever in a very short time. Now, the idea which the old doctors had, that a person with a fever must avoid over eating, was also perfectly sound. They say, for instance, that the nurse should make up her mind what the sick person ought to eat and then give him just about half as much as she thinks the sick person ought to have. And thus, you see there is very little feeding done, and the system has a chance to get rid of this effete matter; it is a subconscious recognition, apparently, of the truth that it is effete matter which causes the disease.

We are further informed that it is very important to regulate the bowels, and we notice that in a case of typhoid fever, diarrhoea is always found accompanying the fever. The reason why this is so is the fact that the fever is caused by the accumulation of effete matter, and the diarrhoea helps to eliminate this, but in a case of typhoid fever, there is so much being disgorged through the bowels, not simply what is there, but there is a lot of this poison being poured into the bowels and it is eventually disgorged. There is danger, sometimes of the bowels ulcerating or bursting; in this case, therefore, we must continue to get all of the effete matter out; and also go about it slowly; don't let the bowels disgorge too much; keep them under control; however, allow the accumulated effete matter to escape, as this is the only way by which the trouble may be cured.

Now, all diseases which are accompanied by fevers are due in whole, or in part, to the accumulation of effete matter in the system and the fever is an effort on the part of nature to get rid of that trouble. Consequently, the way to treat diseases accompanied by fever is to get rid of effete matter. Any way that will accomplish this, any method, rather, that will lead to the realization of this end, will cure the disease. No matter what it may be, it will be found beneficial, and this was the foundation of the old idea that the way to cure these troubles was first to give the patient a cathartic; the idea was to put him on a purgative treatment until the bowels were purged out and then go to work and treat the fever afterwards. While this was right in theory, the practice was not very good; it was decidedly a harsh method to get rid of effete matter in the tissues, by giving a person black pills and calomel, as their action was simply to gather up the liquids of the system and thus, by robbing the system of its liquids, to flush the colon so to speak; that is really the method the cathartic employs, and of course, the method is a cure because what you really want is to eliminate the poison from the cells, to clean out the tissues and pour it into the bowels and, of course, you have got to have the bowels eliminate it, but you need not be in any way uneasy but what the bowels will evacuate the poison if it comes into them.

The presence of diarrhoea is always found to accompany fevers when the fever has reached a very great height.

Another thing which you must bear in mind in treating a disease of this type, is the fact that bilious troubles should be left alone. There is no greater fallacy than that you have to work the bile off. Whenever you get too much bile in the system it will work itself off.

There is one type of diarrhoea known among physicians which is called bilious diarrhoea, which is caused by accumulation of bile until it causes a diarrhoea to set in. Now, if you let that diarrhoea alone and don't try to check it, why it will run on until all the effete matter is driven from the system. After the bowels are cleaned out, then for two

65

or three days, the patient will pass pure bile. We know this by our own experience. We have passed more than two quarts of pure and unadulterated bile without any trace of anything else, thus we know this is true.

When you get bilious, therefore, you have really accumulated the natural purgative of the system; bile is the purgative which nature has provided, and when you get sufficiently bilious, it is truly impossible to retain any effete matter in your system, or, at least in the bowels; they will be cleaned out; that is really the natural method of flushing the colon. It is the bile that carries it all out and when everything else is carried out, then the bile will pass away. There is nothing in the world so beneficial for cleaning out the system as a real, first class, full grown case of bilious diarrhoea. It will do more good than all the doctors in Chicago can do for eliminating the effete matter from the system. In many instances this condition is due to accumulation of fecal matter in the bowels, though, of course, generally speaking, the difficulty is due to starch poison, but sometimes the difficulty is due to the accumulation of fecal matter in the system. If so, fasting will be found to cure it. Whenever fasting cures one, it is because that condition is due to the accumulation of fecal matter in the bowels, and by fasting, we thus cease to feed this condition any further, and thus when we have eliminated the effete matter which was there to begin with, we find that we are all right, the system perfectly cleaned up.

One other point which we must touch on here, though it does not naturally come under this head, is the nefarious iniquity of using salt. There is nothing in the world so detrimental to the health as salt, that is, inorganic salt, which we buy in the stores, such as is employed in the ordinary seasoning of food. Inorganic salt is in its very nature a disrupting force. We take cucumbers, or other food, for that matter, and soak them in brine. Why do we pickle them? To keep them from decaying. Now, the natural course would be for these green vegetables to disintegrate in time after reaching a certain point, and then they will decay. We employ salt because it will separate the organic salt in the fruits or vegetables, and by so doing, will prevent the natural decay. As this salt becomes inorganic, it has the tendency when taken into the system, of disrupting all the organic arrangement of the body. There is nothing in the world so undesirable as the use of mineral salt. In every way, it not only has this effect on the foods, but when we take it into the system, it acts upon our food there and upon the salts which are accumulated in the system; it prevents the elimination of carbon dioxide and the other poisons of the system, and the eliminants of the system are the organic salts of sodium, potassium, calcium, magnesium, phosphorus and silicon. By the use of inorganic salt these organic salts are disorganized, becoming inorganic and cease to eliminate, and on the contrary, they begin to separate and break up and they present the tissue building, so that there is nothing in the world so detrimental to the health as the use of inorganic salt: in fact, if a single grain of salt is taken with an entire meal, it has that effect to the extent that you use it. Of course, it is better to use a small quantity of salt than to use a large quantity, nevertheless the use of salt in any sense, is decidedly undesirable.

You ask me, then, what are we to do? Is it not a fact that we have to have salt: that the system requires it? Yes, but it is organic salt which the system requires, and this is found in vegetables and not in mineral form. Man never was intended to eat anything that was taken out of the ground. His real diet is composed of those plants which are adapted to his use, never animal or mineral food. He can use animal food, however, much better than he can mineral food. Don't employ minerals in your food; that mineral is the natural food of plants, and plants are the natural food of animals; therefore, get all your salt out of plants.

Now, if you eat cereals and nuts and certain vegetables and get salt in this way, it is always organic, provided you don't make it inorganic by cooking. It will also be noticed that the diet of uncooked food does not require the salt that a diet of cooked food requires. When you acquire the habit of eating uncooked food, particularly if you eat cereals, fruits, and nuts, you will not want salt. Salt is mainly required in eating meat and things that grow under ground. The appetite for salt comes in this way and also when we are eating cooked food.

Now, it may occur to you that animals require salt; that they have to be salted at regular intervals or they get in a bad state of health. This is true, but remember that the domestic animal is given only such food as his keepers will provide him, to a great extent; he cannot have the proper kind of food. The result is he does not get the salt in its organic form, that he requires, and the substitute for this is provided in the mineral salt. Also the animal eats a large quantity of food, his food is raw and consequently the salt that he eats does not do so much harm. Remember, the animal will perhaps have salt once or twice a week; he will eat a handful of salt or less; horses and cows will eat less than a handful of salt once a week, or less. At the same time, they will eat fifty ears of corn in a day, and the result is the effect of the salt in this amount of food is not so bad because there is so much food that it is not disorganized; also because of the plainness and simplicity of their diet, it does not have this bad effect. Furthermore, the animal is much more coarsely organized and does not suffer so much from those effects and he does not get in his food the organic salt. The wild animal also at certain times wants to go to a salt lick and get salt, because in the wild state his diet largely consists of grass, bushes, etc., and he does not have an opportunity to select the fine, choice diet that the man has. But for the man who is able to get the proper diet, diet containing salt in the organic form, he should never touch inorganic or mineral salt in any way. Mineral substances are the natural food for plants; vegetable substances the natural food for man.

L E S S O N   O N

S U G G E S T I O N

The various methods of Suggestion may be classified as

FIRST: Auto Suggestion; that is to say when suggestion is offered in your own mind.

SECOND: Suggestion when offered by another.

THIRD: Telepathic Suggestion.

FOURTH: Larvated Suggestion.

FIFTH: Hypnotic Suggestion.

All the various suggestive activities fall under one of these five classifications.

Now, the purpose of Suggestion is to impart to the mind or to form in the mind a picture of the desired condition, inasmuch as the picture formed in mind has the effect of setting up the rate of vibration corresponding to the condition pictured, resulting in a changed vibratory state, expressing itself in an altered condition of the state of the body with reference to health, etc. Auto-Suggestion is employed to enable us to form the desired mental picture. It may be presented in the form either of affirmation or denial. Denials are never desirable, however. When you realize that the purpose of suggestion is to form the picture of a condition, you will then realize that denying a condition is just as efficacious for forming a picture of that condition, as it is to affirm it. When you deny, in your suggestion, a fever, you are making a picture of fever. Now, it does not make any difference what you think about that picture, when the picture is formed, it sets up the vibration corresponding to it, and these states of vibration must express themselves in a condition naturally appertaining to them.

Auto-Suggestion, then, is any aspect of the mind which naturally leads unto the establishment of a corresponding picture. It is a means unto the formation of mental pictures, so that, as a matter of fact, all our lives are practically put in, in giving ourselves auto-suggestions, but the term "AUTO-SUGGESTION" is usually made use of in reference to statements of thought, definitely formulated mental attitudes, for the express purpose of producing these mental pictures and reaching certain conclusions.

In making Auto-Suggestions for the sake of health, we should never try to cure disease. We should, on the contrary, affirm health; make the picture of the condition which we want, not of something which we want to get rid of. In this respect Christian Science is perfectly logical when it denies the reality of disease; that is to say, in affirming that all is good, affirming perfect health and strength and everything of that kind, its members are following along the line of true philosophy, but where they are wrong is in denying certain diseases in order to help them form the picture of the absence of disease. They should follow their methods to their logical result and simply affirm what they want, treating the undesirable condition with silent contempt. If they would do this, they would find themselves able to cure practically all diseases much more easily than they do at the present time and without the disastrous results which sometimes follow the practice of denial. Denial, then is never to be resorted to. Affirmations may, at all times be practiced. Affirmations are necessary, and part of the law of Auto-Suggestion.

It is true Auto-Suggestion is sometimes practiced without the positive affirmations which are very often used. We may go to work and suggest in mind certain conditions taking place, certain processes in the body or anything of that kind, when we do not throw anything like the force and vim into them that you do in making positive affirmation.

On the other hand, in making suggestions, never suggest that you are going to do so and so; that you are going to get well; never make suggestions to take place in the future, because the object of Auto-Suggestion is to form the mental picture; therefore, always form your suggestions in the present tense. Form it in such a way as to induce the picture of a present activity, as health right now, so as to govern the vibration and produce this state of health. Consequently, the injunction in the Scriptures that when you pray for anything, believe that you receive it and you shall receive it, is found to be in strict accordance with psychological law.

Now, Auto-Suggestion is really the key to all the other methods of suggestion. All other methods are simply so many means unto the end of establishing the suggestion in the patient's mind. In the Auto-Suggestion, the suggestive impulse originates within the patient. When suggestion is practiced from the outside, that is, when the physician is giving the suggestion, he gives it in such a way as to cause the patient to repeat it to himself so that the mental picture is produced in his mind. Now, if the patient does not repeat the suggestion to himself, it is absolutely valueless. It can influence him only to the degree that he forms in mind the picture which is suggested by the word of the physician, and to do that he must repeat the suggestion to himself. In other words, the patient must believe what you say in order for it to have any influence on him.

The entire medical practice is made up, as it were, of expedients to produce these pictures in the mind of the patient. All the tactics which are resorted to by the physician to establish confidence on the part of the patient, to make him rely upon the skill of the physician to accomplish his cure — all of these methods are so many tricks to cause the patient to suggest the cure to himself; in other words, to produce the same effect as a strong Auto-Suggestion would produce.

Go where you will, you see this activity in continuous operation, therefore, the physician who would practice suggestion must always manifest confidence himself, because there is nothing so contagious as confidence. If the physician has within himself a doubt of his ability to cure his patient, a doubt of the efficacy of any remedial agent which he may apply, this doubt will make it impossible for the agent to have the desired effect, because it will be impressed upon the mind of the patient so that he will not have the requisite degree of confidence, and therefore, will not repeat the suggestion to himself; will not be cured.

What is LARVATED SUGGESTION? The masked suggestion is practiced whenever a physical agent is administered for the purpose of inspiring confidence in the patient; that is to say, a drug is given not with the expectation of curing the patient with the drug, but simply to establish confidence so that the patient will expect to be cured. He will be in an attitude of expectation and this attitude of expectation will cause him to form the picture of health, will establish the vibration which will heal his body. The use of ninety per cent of the remedial agents, so-called, of the intelligent physician, is simply for the purpose of masking a suggestion. In a case of this kind it is very often highly beneficial to make the patient believe he is taking a very strong agent of some kind; that the medicine is very powerful and you do not know whether he will live through it or not; it is very likely to kill him if it doesn't have exactly the right effect, and remember the patient is expecting relief from the drug and consequently he must think he is getting a very powerful one. A case in point is that of a physician in the South whom we knew personally. He has accomplished a number of very wonderful cures. He has built up a great reputation for successful practice and he says himself, that the cases that have made him, were cases where he did not know what was the matter with his patients and he would leave a bottle of water with the patient, to be measured out and taken and then await developments, and the water has cured the patient and it has built up this physician's reputation. There was a man whose wife had been troubled with

71

sciatica for quite a while. This doctor had treated her, had given her everything the books prescribed, but even though relieved, it would, in a short time, come back. The husband finally came to the doctor and said, "Doctor, my wife is down with that sciatica again and suffering terribly. Can't you do something?" The doctor opened a drawer in his desk, saying, "Well, I hate like thunder to give her these tablets, but I guess I will have to," and he took out three tablets, gave them to the man and said, "You take these home; give one to your wife as soon as you get there. Tell her I said she would get better right straight, but if in half an hour she is not relieved, give the second one and if that doesn't relieve her in half an hour, give the third, and I know the third will cure her. But you tell her I said she would get better right straight after she takes the first." Well the man went home and said to his wife, "Mary, Doc sent you some medicine now that will cure. He said for you to take this tablet and you would get better right away." She took it, suffering terribly. In half an hour she got up, put on her clothes and got supper, and for two years after that never had a touch of sciatica. Her husband was talking to the doctor and said, "Doc, that must have been terribly strong medicine you gave my wife. She has never had a touch of sciatica again. What was it Doc?" and he replied, "Loaf Sugar."

This is a fair sample of the way many physicians practice, although there are not many who have the courage to carry it out the way this doctor did; nevertheless, it will accomplish wonderful results. So many cures have been accomplished by physicians who are simply giving remedies as agents for Larvated Suggestion. When an agent is given that way, the patient believing it to be a strong medicine and having confidence in the use of drugs, it will naturally produce a more powerful picture in mind than could possibly be produced in such persons with any other kind of suggestion. For this reason, it is often the most beneficial method that could be resorted to. People should never be given drugs, but it is very often quite beneficial to give them loaf sugar or starch or flour, or cold water and tell them it is medicine. If they think it is a drug it may have a much more beneficial effect than if they knew what it really is. In the practice of Larvated Suggestion, therefore, we simply use an agent as a means of establishing an Auto-Suggestion in the patient's mind.

In Telepathic Suggestion, we do not speak. It is not something we say or something we do that communicates the suggestion, but it is the thought. The thought is projected from the mind of the physician direct to the mind of the patient. This may be either conscious or unconscious. The most of suggestion of this kind is unconscious. If there is a degree of sympathy between the physician and the patient, there is danger of all the physician's thoughts being communicated to the patient as soon as they enter his mind; consequently if a physician gives up hope of curing his patient he should immediately drop the case. No physician should try to cure a case that he does not believe he can cure, because every time he visits the patient he is projecting the poisonous thought. He is suggesting unconsciously to himself, death, and is consequently building up a picture of death which will, in time, establish the death dealing rhythm and, of course, the patient is murdered by the skepticism of his doctor. But again, we have silent suggestion which is resorted to for the express purpose of establishing the picture in the mind of the patient. That is, we may think thoughts for the purpose of acting as suggestions. In other words, we practice suggestion, only we do not speak it. We think the suggestion silently instead of speaking it, and this is just as powerful, in fact, more so, than the spoken suggestion. The practice of Christian Scientists in sitting by the side of the patient and realizing health for him, without saying anything, without talking, but practicing the Eddy Silent Method, as it is called, silently realizing health and truth for the patient, is based upon this principle. As we formulate in mind a picture of the patient in that condition which we desire him to realize, we in this way, establish that state of mind, we establish in him that consciousness, consequently we are practicing bona fide suggestion. We do this by sitting by his bedside or we may practice it at a considerable distance, in fact, thousands of miles, in some cases, the method being perfectly the same.

The possibility for telepathic suggestion unconsciously, even to the one who is making the suggestion, that is to say, the capacity of thought for traveling from the mind which projected it, to another mind, without the will or desire of either party concerned, makes it very dangerous for sick people to be in the environment of those who do not understand the law and who are not living in harmony with healthful thoughts, etc. It is, for this reason that it is much better for patients to be treated in sanitariums where they will be separated from their friends, from everybody as nearly as possible, who will be thinking adverse to their recovery. It is also best that the world should not know of their condition, particularly if they are in a critical state, because if it be known, there will be danger of the thought of the world coming to the patient, in spite of everything that can be done.

Hypnotic Suggestion is the same as the last described, with the exception that the patient, when hypnotized, is unable to refuse the suggestion. In other forms of suggestion, his judgment is active. He may accept or reject the suggestion at will, but when he is hypnotized it is utterly impossible for him to exercise any such selective judgment. He must accept whatever suggestion comes from the hypnotist and, accepting it, he must repeat it, and thus it forms the mental picture which will express itself in vibration. In a word, when hypnotized, you do not have a word to say in regard to the pictures that are hung up in your mental picture gallery. The hypnotist decides this for himself, and for this reason a hypnotic suggestion is much more powerful than the ordinary suggestion. It cannot be gainsaid at all; you believe it; you cannot help believing it because your intellectual activity and everything is governed by the will of the hypnotist, consequently it is more powerful in its effects on the physical body though, of course, detrimental to the will of the patient. The hypnotist, however, is not suggesting by what he says, but what he thinks. Every thought which comes into his mind is immediately projected to the mind of the patient. He knows exactly what is in the mind of the operator; knowing this he acts upon it. It is, therefore, highly important that the hypnotist should have absolute control of his thinking while he is hypnotizing his patient, because it is not what he says, but what he thinks that really constitutes the suggestion, and when the suggestion is formed, has gone into the mind of the patient, has formulated a corresponding mental picture, it is then, of course, too late to remedy the evil, if it be an evil which is formed.

Suggestion, then, is the application of thought either expressed in words or not so expressed, for the purpose of formulating a mental picture of the desired result in the mind of the patient — Auto-Suggestion when it is formed by the patient himself at first hand; in other forms of suggestion it comes from another. External Suggestion is a means unto the formation of Auto-Suggestion within the patient. The suggestion is a definite statement which, in its nature, has the effect of establishing the corresponding picture.

In one sense all suggestion is by affirmation; that is to say, the statement conveys with it a certain picture; it thus affirms that picture. But denials, while affirming the picture, may be denying the very thing which they affirm; that is to say, they may deny in an intellectual sense, that certain conditions exist, nevertheless, they are forming the picture of that condition.

We may speak of ourselves, in practicing Auto-Suggestion, in the first person, or in the second person. A very good way to practice Auto-Suggestion is to give yourself a talking to once in a while; talk to yourself in the second person. That is quite a good way.

But in any event, Suggestion is a means unto the formation of pictures of a desired condition and it is, therefore, to its use as an agent unto mental picturing that all the efficacy of Suggestive Therapeutics is due.

LESSON ON

MAGNETIC HEALING

The basis of Suggestive Therapeutics, it should be borne in mind, is the ability to direct and control the activity of the magnetic current within the organism of the patient by reason of the influence of the imagination acting thereon, likewise the ability to control the Astral energy through the mental pictures which are formed in the mind of the patient by reason of the suggestion offered. It will be seen, therefore, that in a general sense, particularly in the treatment of functional diseases, the principal utility of suggestion is the influence which it exercises upon the magnetism or vital current of the patient. Any other method, which will control the magnetic current of the patient or which will supply the healer's magnetism will be likewise efficacious.

Suggestive Therapeutics is, in reality the direction of those forces within the body of the patient, through the instrumentality of a suggestion offered to his mind.

Magnetic Healing is the application of the magnetism of the healer to the body of the patient in such a way as to direct the circulation of the patient's magnetic current to restore equilibrium in the circulatory activity of the same, to control its distribution and, in some instances, the supplying of the magnetism of the healer direct to the body of the patient for the purpose of acting in place of his own. This latter method is particularly resorted to in cases where the patient lacks tone, where he is weak — constitutional treatment, in other words. Even in local treatment, however, it may be found necessary to magnetize the organ and local nerve center in order that it may perform its work until the system has had time to recuperate its own energies.

The oldest method of Magnetic Healing was by passes. The passes are resorted to for the purpose of directing the circulation of the vital force. The rationale of magnetic passes lies in the fact that you may control your own magnetism wherever it may be. If it is in the body of the patient, it is just as much under your control as it is when in your own body. By magnetizing the patient's body, in such a way that your own magnetism becomes mixed, as it were, with his, and directing the circulation of this magnetism, which you have placed in his body, you are, in this way, able to direct the circulation of his own. The passes are, therefore, made either with contact, that is when the fingers touch the body, or without contact, when they are made at a slight distance from the body. In either case, you must keep a current of magnetism streaming through the ends of your fingers, entering the body of the patient and blending with his own magnetic current. Now, you should begin with the brain of the patient and gradually, while maintaining the mind in a state of deep concentration, draw the hands down in the same way, continually keeping the picture in mind, drawing his magnetic force down to the plane where the weakness is, where you want the magnetism and even below; thus keep the current going through it until you have concentrated all the magnetism you can. Then as you raise your hands, be careful to turn them so that the back of the hand will be exposed to the patient, also bringing them up with a curved motion going outward for a while and then going back so that they are brought together again over the top of his head. In this way you will not draw the magnetism upward while you are raising the hands. If you allow the arms to be near the patient you will have the effect of drawing the current backward; then repeat the passes, drawing it down again until the treatment is over. In this way you will be establishing the circulation in that part of the body.

The passes in this way act in precisely the same way upon the nerve currents that massaging an organ, or the application of mechano-therapy-manipulation to a muscle, does in stimulating the circulation of the blood. You have turned the circulation of the nerve force into that particular part of the body. You have charged it with the magnetic force and it will continue to flow there for some time afterwards, and the energy that you put there will in the meantime have accomplished its work.

Do not be deceived with the idea that the relief which follows a magnetic treatment is permanent — that is to say, that a chemical change has taken place and that the symptom is permanently cured because it has disappeared. The relief which usually follows a magnetic treatment is due to the fact that artificial stimulus has been supplied to the nerve centers. They are able to do their work much more effectively than they did before, but they are doing this work with a force other than their own. After a while, in the course of time, it will be discovered that the special stimulus has been exhausted, consequently the patient will be in the same condition as before. The magnetic treatments, therefore, must be continued for some time after the patient is apparently cured, until the defect has been removed, and the patient has had a chance to accumulate the necessary amount of energy unto the successful performance of the work.

In a word, a permanent cure is one thing; the relief of disease symptoms by magnetic treatment is quite another thing. In some cases you may want to give simply a general constitutional treatment, that is, to send the magnetic current through the body. There may not be any particular local trouble you wish to relieve, but you may find it expedient to stimulate the circulation of the Prana throughout the system. In this way you should make your passes from the top of the head down to the soles of the feet, even below, swooping downward, and remember, do not make the passes in jerks, make them in one continuous motion. Let there be one continuous movement from the top of the head to the soles of the feet, swinging the hands backward, swinging the arms around, bringing them up to the top of the head. In this way you will give a continuous current.

Remember, also, there are certain directions in which the vital forces circulate in the body and you should follow that natural course, so as to quicken and stimulate the circulation, in the regular way, not going contrary to the regular course of things; consequently if you want to treat a disease which is a manifestation of a weakness in the cerebro-spinal nervous system, you want to follow that course, that is to say, you want to make the passes down the spinal column until you come to where those nerves branch off from the spinal cord. Whenever you reach that point, you should swing your hands along that nerve, so as to reach the organ; that is the proper way to make the passes.

If you want to stimulate the entire cerebro-spinal nervous system, bring your hands down the spinal cord close together, and down to the sacral plexus and then down either limb and to the ends of the toes. It is a very good way in giving treatments of this kind, to place the patient on the table, face downward, and then come down the spinal cord, following the course of the cerebro-spinal nerves.

If giving passes by contact, it will be found expedient in many instances, to have the patient nude and to press rather firmly on the tissue, with the fingers, while making the passes. However, you can give this kind of treatment through the clothing (though it is a little more difficult) providing the patient does not have on any silk. If wearing silk garments, it will be found very difficult to give a magnetic treatment. You may, of course, if you are performing Spiritual or Divine Healing, accomplish a great deal through the clothing even if the patient have on silk; but silk is an absolute insulation to Physical magnetism and the Astral magnetism, which contains the Prana, cannot get through it as well as through other garments, but, where possible, it will be found best to treat the nude

77

body. For this reason it is very often expedient to pretend to practice massage while practicing magnetic healing. Massage or Osteopathy, Chiropractic or Mechano-therapy are frequently excellent blinds to use in carrying on the practice of magnetic healing.

It should be borne in mind also, that any disturbance in the circulation of a nerve will effect all the organs and muscles which are supplied by that nerve, consequently where the vertebrae press upon the nerve passing between them, it will be impossible for the proper amount of nervous stimuli to pass through that nerve.

The practice of Osteopathy and Chiropractic are, therefore, founded upon a truth. In order to restore the state of health permanently, it will be found necessary to relieve that pressure. This may be done either by mechanical manipulation as those systems do, or it may be done by the application of magnetism, stimulus to the nerves which will so act as to relieve the pressure, by causing the muscles to move and separate those vertebrae which have been pinching the nerve. However, the mechanical adjustment will give relief, although it is undoubtedly better in the long run to have the adjustment gradually accomplished through the activity of the magnetic force, than to have it accomplished suddenly through mechanical adjustment. The reason for this is that had the nerves been acting properly, had the proper degree of stimulus been received and had the muscles properly responded to the same, no such condition would ever have existed. The adjustment is required only by reason of the fact that the body is not properly responding to this nervous stimulus. Now, to apply a mechanical force is to relieve the muscles of the duty of responding to nervous stimulus, consequently, to make them less amenable to such influence. It is, therefore, better to have the adjustment accomplished through the concentration of magnetic force than through the application of mechanical adjustment.

The principle which I wish you to bear in mind is this: In applying magnetism you must follow along the natural course of that nerve circulation — never go against it. Consequently in stimulating the cerebro-spinal circulation, you must act along the course of the cerebro-spinal nerves. It should be borne in mind that, generally speaking, the cerebro-spinal nerves control the human structure, the shell, as it were, the bodily organization, while the organs, the functional part of the body, the vital activities, are controlled by the sympathetic nervous system. Always bear this in mind; never try to treat the latter troubles through the cerebro-spinal nerves, but work through the sympathetic nerves. Bear in mind that the sympathetic nervous system centers in the solar plexus. Any weakness of the sympathetic nervous system is due to the fact that there is not a sufficient quantity of nerve stimuli flowing to the Solar Plexus. You cannot, therefore, remedy a weakness of the sympathetic nervous system

78

as long as the Solar Plexus is weak. The first thing to do then, is to stimulate the circulation of the Prana in the Solar Plexus, so that it is charged, as it were, then act upon the sympathetic nerve, which runs from the Solar Plexus to the particular organ which you wish to treat. If you do not know just the direction, make your passes in such a way as to go from the Solar Plexus to that particular organ the best way you can, and they will find the nerve which will lead there.

Another way in which you may treat the weaknesses of the body is by always remembering that there are two currents, the electrical and the magnetic. These two currents are found on all the planes of nature, in each of the principles. Bear in mind that Prana is both electrical and magnetic. The electrical force is generated in the left hemisphere of the brain; the nerve currents crossing, it consequently, flows down the right side of the body. The spinal column or spinal cord is double, having an electrical and magnetic side. Those nerves which branch off from the right side of the spinal column, the three large pairs of nerves, are electrical; the left side, on the contrary, is magnetic. Each of these pairs of nerves is double, there being a sensory and a motor nerve and these divide into the diverse branches. Therefore, if you find your patient is lacking in magnetism, make your passes from the spinal cord to the left over the left side of the body. If he is lacking in electricity, make them from the spinal cord to the right side of the body. A very good way to do this is to make them down the right arm and the right leg, or the left arm and the left leg, as the case may be, but you may make them over the body in general — the particular side of the body which you wish to treat. However, it should be borne in mind that different sections of the cerebro-spinal nervous system are controlled by different plexuses and the particular plexus which controls that organ should be stimulated, therefore, if you want to govern or control the nerves in a certain part of the body, make your passes in such a way as to draw the current as far down as the plexus, below the one controlling those nerves. Remember, the head and face are controlled by the medulla oblongata direct, that is to say, the nerves of the head and face radiate from the medulla oblongata and do not go down the spinal column below that.

The shoulders and the upper chest are governed by the Cervical Plexus immediately between the shoulders where they join the neck lying on either side of the spinal cord.

The lower chest and back are governed by the Dorsal Plexus where the shoulders join the back proper, that is to say, at the lower extremity of the shoulder. The Lumbar Region or Spinal Region, properly speaking, is, of course, governed by the lumbar plexus.

The pelvic cavity, together with the sex organs, the hips and the lower limbs, are governed by the sacral plexus. This, in fact, governs the entire sacral region and lies on either side of the spinal column at its lower extremity. All the nerves which have not already branched off from the spinal column, branch off there. It may be found by examining the point where the hips join the backbone — right there is where you will find the Sacral Plexus and that is the point, the positive pole, so to speak, of the nervous circulation in all that part of the body.

Remember, that the positive pole is the plexus, and the nerve center, which you wish to control, is the negative pole, therefore, place your positive hand, which if you wish to treat electrically, should be the right, if magnetically, the left — place this positive hand over the plexus controlling the nerve centers, which you wish to treat; place the negative hand over the weakened part, the nerve center where you want the current to go, and then concentrate and the current will be established and flow from your positive hand through the plexus and through the nerve center into the negative hand. As long as you keep your hands there and keep up this concentration, the current will flow, and you treat it in precisely the same way you would treat with an electric battery. If you wish to strengthen the plexus, then you proceed in a different way; you place your negative hand over the plexus which you want to treat; your positive hand you place either along the spinal cord at the base of the brain and gradually draw down to the negative hand with passes, thus directing the current down, or else you may place it at the base of the brain, and then, by concentration, make a current go down through the spinal cord. You place your hand, that is, your positive hand, upon the Solar Plexus and your negative hand over the region of the nerve center which you wish to treat, if you want to treat the sympathetic nerves in this way by stimulating the activity of certain organs; or else you may place your right hand on the patient's head, and left or negative hand, on the Solar Plexus and treat in this way. In some instances you may place the right positive hand on the Solar Plexus, charging it direct and with the left hand clasp the patient by one of his hands so as to close the circuit, and thus impart the magnetism in this way.

Remember, now, that magnetism is physical or vital as the case may be, the physical being the electric-magnetic force of the Etheric Double and the same as electricity; the vital being the electro-magnetic life force which acts through the Astral Body. In either case, however, it is no higher than the Astral. It is closely analogous to the sex force, in fact, it is an aspect of the sex force, particularly Astral vital magnetism. This is generated in the organ of vitativeness and amativeness and if you want to give your patient more magnetism, you can very often accomplish it through the stimulation of those organs.

In healing it is, therefore, discovered that the magnetism of

the healer is imparted to the body of the patient, and he is beneficial in just the degree to which he imparts his own magnetism to his
patient's body and the purer the magnetism is, the freer from detrimental influences, of course, the better will be its effect. Whatever
is the condition of the healer — physical condition, we mean, that
will be imparted to the organism of the patient, through his magnetism.

Suggestion is employed for the purpose of directing the patient's
own magnetism.

Magnetic Healing is the magnetism of a healer imparted to the
body of the patient, either for the purpose of acting as a substitute
for his own magnetism or else as the means of directing that magnetism.

L E S S O N   O N

S E X U A L   H E A L I N G

In the study of the diverse healing or therapeutic agents presented in the human constitution, it is peculiar to observe that no
one, apparently, has recognized the great healing potency resident in
the polarity of the sex principle. Far more efficacious than simple
magnetic healing is this sex principle. We mean the application of the
sex principle as such. It is, in fact, the application of the law of
polarity to magnetic healing, magnetic healing dealing, as it were,
with magnetism in the united or blended state without reference to the
pole to which it belongs, whether it be electrical or magnetic. A much
greater percentage of diseases, however, are caused by an improper
polarization of this electro-magnetic force. What we mean is that if
we get too electrical or too magnetic as the case may be, there are
certain diseases which result directly from this condition. Amongst
the diseases which are caused by an excessively electrical condition,
may be included all forms of fever, cholera, cholera morbus, diarrhoea
and everything of that kind. All diseases indicated by a looseness of
the bowels, in fact, are due to an excessively electrical condition.

Now, it will be borne in mind by the student that in previous
lessons, it has been indicated that those bowel complaints were due to
the fact that the system had been clogged up with effete matter, and
that is true, but that might cause all the flowing or running of the
bowels and it is an excessively electrical condition of the system
which causes the expulsion from the system of those waste products.

It should be borne in mind, therefore, that the natural cure for
a clogged up system is to induce an electrical condition. If you treat
the system with magnetism, you will make it worse. By employing the
electrical pole, the masculine, electro-magnetic energy, it will be
seen that you will almost immediately bring about this change which will
expel the poisonous substances from the system through the healing
current, manifesting itself in a discharge from the bowels.

82

Also, it should be borne in mind that the accumulation of effete matter has a tendency to establish an electrical condition which will, in turn, expel it from the system. This is a wise provision which nature has made. When the system becomes clogged and loaded with effete matter, this effete matter produces an electrical condition, and the electrical condition expels the matter from the body. Consequently, if let alone the accumulation will expel itself and thus bring relief, providing the accumulation is not so great that the electrical condition becomes too powerful, producing a violent diarrhoea, in which case, of course, it must be checked by the application of magnetic force to neutralize this excessively electrical condition.

Fevers are electrical in the same way and manifest the electrical heat-generating principle which destroys effete matter and thus brings relief. Fever or any other electrical condition is the natural destructive agent and therefore, natural curative agent for these accumulations, though if it become too high and it is found expedient to cool off the fever, it should be borne in mind that the remedy is magnetism; if electrical force be employed it will kill the patient in a very short time.

Healing, therefore, by one who does not understand the law of polarity, is very dangerous, just as the practice of electro-therapeutics, by one who does not understand this polarizing law, becomes exceedingly dangerous.

We know cholera to be an electrical condition. One of the facts which illustrate this point to perfection was brought forward in Naples during the cholera epidemic quite a number of years ago. There was a steel weight, weighing one hundred pounds, which was held suspended by magnetic attraction between the points of a horse shoe magnet which was suspended from the ceiling in the Gallery of Science. This had been there for over a hundred years, the magnetism in the magnet being strong enough to maintain it in its state of suspension. The cholera was raging. All Italy was prostrate. The entire army was there and they undertook to handle the sick. People were dying in the streets, the fever raging everywhere. It was as if a pall had fallen over Naples. All at once there was an earthquake. Instantaneously the steel weight fell to the floor, the fever cooled on every patient in Naples and the epidemic was over. What is the explanation? The atmosphere was intensely electrical, everything was electrical and consequently the air had the cholera; everything had the cholera, and it affected the people. They had all taken on an intensely electrical condition. Cholera was, therefore, raging. From some cause, planetary influence, perhaps, there was a tremendous influx of magnetic force which charged the whole air, rendering it magnetic. The result was, the steel became charged with magnetism, and therefore, became for time being a magnet. As two magnets are mutually repellant, the magnetic attraction ceased; it was driven from the magnet to the floor, each repelling the other and the atmosphere becoming magnetic, the people were charged with magnetism from this magnetic atmosphere, the magnetic current neutralizing the electrical current, and thus the cholera was expelled from them, the fever left them.

The earthquake was, of course, due to the proximity of the volcano, Vesuvius, and the magnetic current which filled the air and the earth and everything, awakened the electro-magnetic force in the volcano, which produced the earthquake.

This, therefore, illustrates to perfection the principle that cholera is due to an electrical condition of the organism, and anything which will induce a magnetic condition will accomplish a cure. It also explains why some people are far more susceptible to cholera infection than others, being more electrical, and therefore, having less magnetic resistance to be overcome in order to establish the electrical cholera condition.

The healer who is successful in treating cholera is, consequently, the magnetic person, and the person who is intensely magnetic will find it comparatively safe to treat and nurse cholera patients, as such a person has so much magnetism that it is difficult for it to be overcome. The treatment, then, for cholera must be magnetic, not electric.

Now, among those diseases which are caused by an intense, an excessively magnetic condition, are all forms of cold, catarrh, consumption, hay fever and all that type of diseases, although, of course, the remote cause is the accumulation of starch poison in the system, but that condition will manifest itself in those diseases, the immediate cause being an intensely magnetic condition of the body. The magnetic condition causes the expulsion in this way, and if you will look at it properly you will see that the magnetic influence is one of the laws which Nature has devised to relieve those conditions, it being thus the manifestation of the Great Wisdom which has been shown in causing the accumulation of effete matter, and in this case produce a magnetic condition which will expel it from the system.

If you wish to treat these troubles in such a way as to stop the symptom instead of allowing the elimination in the ordinary way, or if the elimination is too rapid — if you want, in a word, to stop the symptom as it manifests, the treatment should be electrical, not magnetic, unless you want to aggravate it.

Everything which manifests itself by choking or constipation of the bowels, is also a magnetic condition and in order to induce a looseness of the bowels, electrical force should be applied, the electrical force having the tendency to relax the muscles and consequently allow the expulsion of the excrementory matter, while magnetic force has a tendency to contract and, therefore, retain it.

Now, it should be borne in mind that heat is a mode of electrical

vibration, while cold is a mode of magnetic vibration. Wherever cold is
applied it produces the magnetic influence and heat the electrical. It
will, therefore, be seen at once that the practice of using injections
of warm water into the colon for relieving a constipated state of the
bowels, is strictly in harmony with the electro-magnetic principles
which we have been applying all the way through. In a word, it is a means
of imparting the electrical influence to the colon. Cold water would
impart a magnetic influence; consequently, cold water is a perfect cure
for a discharge, and it has been discovered that even in the menstrual
discharge when it goes beyond the proper time, when there is danger of
the patient bleeding to death, by immersing the body in a bath of cold
water, the worst kind of a discharge, the most alarming, can be stopped in
a few minutes. This is the application of the same principle.

Now, by using the magnetic principle in electro-therapeutics,
that is to say, the negative pole of the battery, you can produce the
same effect, in a way, or the positive pole for the electrical influence,
as the case may be.

But now, to come to the application of these principles to Sexual
Healing. The masculine sex energy is electrical, what is commonly termed
positive, while the feminine is magnetic, or negative, as it is usually
expressed. The positive or electrical force is generated in the left
hemisphere of the brain and passed in currents down the right side of
the body; the feminine or magnetic principle, is generated in the right
hemisphere of the brain and passed down the left side of the body. In
the male, of course, the electrical principle very greatly predominates
over the magnetic, while in the female, the magnetic greatly predominates over the electrical; but we find in the human family, various
degrees in the proportional manifestation of these activities. It should
always be borne in mind that mankind is largely the product of those
forces. We see a person who is excessively electrical, so much so that the
feminine principle is practically absent. The result is, he is dried up,
as it were; the skin becomes hard and dry. There is no brightness in the
eyes; the heart becomes hard and the joints stiff; the step is halting;
there is no life to speak of. He becomes jaundiced in a way. Now, if we
look at this case properly we see that the man is intensely electrical
and is dying for want of the magnetic principle. In such a case let him
fall in love; let him particularly get married, and it will be found that
in a comparatively short time this condition will have entirely left
him. His flesh fills out, his eyes brighten, his complexion clears, his
entire being is pulsating with new life. What are the facts in the case?
He has simply drawn from his wife the magnetism which he required to
restore the equilibrium; he has obtained equilibrium by reason of feeding on his wife's magnetism and for this reason marriage has been, for
him, very desirable. It is not anything like so much in sexual intercourse as in the magnetic exchange which is secured by reason of the

85

society of the wife, which benefits the married man in this particular way.

How many people have noticed the fact that old bachelors become crusty and harsh in their ways, and it has been discovered, therefore, that generally speaking, love between the sexes has been advantageous. The reason why old bachelors become what they are is because of the excessively electrical condition, which becomes developed within them and they require the magnetic influence. On the other hand, old maidishness among women is due to an excessively magnetic influence. The reason why married women do not become old maidish is because they are drawing the electrical principle from their husbands, and at the same time giving off their magnetic principle to them. Thus the equilibrium is maintained.

Now, when a woman is transmitting magnetism to a man who is starving for it, if she has an over abundance of magnetism, it is good for her, but if she has not, then it is not so desirable, and vice versa. The principle of love and marriage is that interchange of the electro-magnetic principle between the sexes.

Now, this principle manifests itself in certain characteristics. We see children who cannot be still, they are "fidgity," and all the time full of mischief, in many instances. The bad boy, the mischievous child, is not so because he is constitutionally mean. It is really from a superabundance of life, energy, sex energy, in a way, because the sex energy manifests long before the time of puberty, in fact, during all life, but this differentiation becomes very strong after puberty, and boys of this type and men, are such because of the superabundance of electrical energy. Fast girls and women, on the other hand are such because of the superabundance of magnetic energy. If they could get rid of this they would become normal. The normal type is where the equilibrium is properly maintained. The abnormalities are due to an excessive condition one way or the other. Now if they are married, or if they are in love, there is then an interchange of these principles which brings the relief required, or in any event, allows them to transmit to the beloved object the over abundance of energy and at the same time to draw from that one the other element, so as to maintain the state of equilibrium. Artists, painters, etc., transmit a great deal of their sexual energy to their work, etc.

Now, what we mean by Sexual Healing, is that the principle which is unconsciously applied in marriage and love may be consciously and deliberately applied in the practice of therapeutics. What we mean is that those persons who find themselves suffering from a superabundance of sex energy, may employ it in the healing of disease. Thus they may get rid of it. However, it must be borne in mind that to do this properly, in those cases, men should be healers of women and women healers of men. Of course, a case of "Lost Manhood" should be treated by a man because in such case there is a lack of the electrical principle, and in women, cases of sexual impotency should be treated by women because there is a weakness of the magnetic principle. Generally speaking, sexual disorders should be treated by the same kind of magnetism which the patient may possess, because in such cases, it is due to a weakness of the normal principle; but there are, of course, exceptions even in sexual disorders but in the main it will be found better for men to have female healers and for women to have male healers. Particularly in treating those diseases which, in their nature, indicate an abundance of the electrical over the magnetic force in male patients, women should be resorted to, to impart the magnetic principle. On the other hand, where the disease indicates an over abundance of magnetism, the electrical principle should be imparted to maintain the state of equilibrium. This practice will be applying the strictly natural principle to the treatment of disease. It will be extremely rational in its character because it will be removing the cause, it will be supplying the natural defect, and at the same time it will relieve the healers of the superabundance of sex energy which they, themselves possess.

There is absolutely no question that the susceptibility of girls to seduction is due to their intense femininity, or the intense magnetic state. There is a demand for an outflowing, a demand absolutely that this magnetic force should escape and in such cases they are easily induced to commit sexual crimes. Many girls become prostitutes for no other reason than the fact that they have a superabundance of magnetic force which must express itself in some way, and society has not seen a way to provide a means for this, consequently they yield. The dissipation and sexual perversion of men are due also to an excessively electrical condition, and by the development of this method of healing, there will be provided a natural avenue of escape for all of this energy.

In this way it will be seen that Nature has really provided remedies for all the ills of life, if we only knew where to look for them. Let the fast woman and amorous man, therefore, engage in the practice of healing and let them heal persons of the opposite sex, and they will find the avenue of escape. This may sound strange to the reader, to be recommended, in cases of excessive voluptuousness, or amorousness, or wantonness to go into the practice among members of the opposite sex, but this is exactly what is requisite. In this way they will get rid of that force, that energy which is prompting them along the lines of sexual excess.

The sexual pervert is, therefore, simply one who has an over abundance of sex energy, which is improperly directed. Those cases, however, where women contract an unnatural passion for members of their own sex are due to the fact that they are not normal women; that is to say, not magnetic, but are intensely electrical, and are demanding magnetism. They must get rid of the electrical force, consequently they are drawn to women, and this trouble can be relieved by their going into the healing business and healing other women, having women for their patients instead of having men patients. Likewise, men who have an unnatural inclination toward other men may have the condition relieved by treating men because in such cases, they are feminine, in a way. They are full of the feminine principle, or magnetism. Thus the allusion to certain characters as being effeminated, is correct, if we understand by this term not weakness, but simply an abundance of magnetism, rather than electrical force; and the "Mannish" woman is such because she has more electrical force than magnetic.

The great difficulty has been that Western Doctors have failed to realize the two principles and their operation throughout all nature. Now, the Yogis understand this perfectly and a great portion of their philosophy is built up upon this principle of the twofold sex differentiation in nature. We learn, in their philosophy and that of the Sankhya school, likewise, that there are two currents which pass down from the brain. The spinal cord is really represented by a number of figure "8's," one resting over the other. These figures will, therefore, represent two hollow tubes, one on either side, with also a place between where they come together, and it should be understood that that also, is tubular. Now, down the right side of this, down the right tube, flows the electrical force, down the left side, the magnetic. What we term the electrical or magnetic force, they term the "Gunas," and the two Gunas flow through the system. They go down until they have gone over the body. They reach the bottom of the spinal cord, the triangular-shaped pocket at the bottom of the spinal cord, the sacral plexus. There the sex energy accumulates; that is to say, that which is not used up by the body in the ordinary vitalizing processes, and by the sexual organs and sexual intercourse, that which does not go to generate the sexual influence, that which is left after all other purposes have been fulfilled, is stored up and coils up in the Serpent, the Kundalini, which remains in that pocket at the bottom. Now, it cannot return the way it came, as this hollow which is between the two, right in the center of the spinal cord, is stopped up by a bony partition which covers the triangular pocket in the sacral plexus. This stopped up or coiled up Kundalini, the Serpent, may however, by certain regular practices be made to strike on the partition as it is raised up, and as you make it rise up and strike there, it will at last, batter away that bony partition and open the way. Then, in time, as it continues to accumulate, by certain Yogi practices, it may be raised up until it reaches the lumbar plexus, when it gives a certain degree of illumination, physical illumination, we will say. Illumination on the physical plane comes from this. When it has risen until it has reached the dorsal plexus, Astral illumination comes. At last, as it reaches the cervical plexus, Mental illumination is the result, and when finally it is brought on up to the Medulla

Oblongata, it there leads to Buddhic illumination, and when finally the Kundalini goes on until it fills the Thousand-Petalled Lotus of the brain, Spiritual illumination comes to us.

We, therefore, find that illumination consists of the drawing up of the Kundalini, through this opening, to the brain. The circuit is from this time restored. The sex force then, when it goes down to the bottom of the spinal cord to the sacral plexus and has nourished the body, is drawn upward and flows back, both poles together. Being now polarized, it flows back to the brain, and this gives Adeptship, Illumination, etc.

It can now be seen why it is so dangerous for any one but celibates to practice those exercises, the design of which is to draw up the Kundalini. They draw the sex force upward, but if this be dissipated, through indulgence, the result will be insanity in every instance. One who does not lead a perfectly chaste life should never think of performing those practices.

It is, consequently by the polarizing of those forces which are ordinarily sent forth to one of the opposite sex, by polarizing them and bringing them back up into our own being, restoring them to the brain, that the regeneration of the body is made possible. The Sexual principle is, therefore, the great healing force of the human organism and should be employed intelligently as a healing agent; but to do this it is necessary to lead a pure life. It is for this reason that celibates are able to do much more effective healing than married men and women or than people who do not lead perfectly chaste lives. If they do not lead lives of perfect purity, they will transmit what force they have, of course, but it will not be anything like as effective — may, in fact, rob them of the energy which they require.

The Sex Energy is generated in the Organ of Amativeness, consequently, to develop this principle in another person, you should apply magnetism to his Organ of Amativenes at the base of the brain. If you want to stimulate magnetism, apply it to the right organ, the one in the right hemisphere of the brain. If you would stimulate electrical force, apply it to the left, and in this way you can stimulate the correct force or principle by stimulating that center, that faculty, which under ordinary conditions will generate that principle within the organism.

If it is inconvenient to treat only members of the opposite sex, for instance, if you want to give both kinds of treatment, both electrical and magnetic, you may accomplish the work by always using the right hand as the positive hand when giving electrical treatments, and the left hand should always be the positive hand when giving magnetic treatments. Also, when stimulating the magnetic force in your patient, place your left or magnetic hand upon the right side of the brain. Your right, or electric hand, if you want to treat the brain, also, should be placed on the left or electrical side; but if you do not wish to do that, if you wish to treat the body, then take the patient's right hand as being the electrical side; if the contrary, use the other hand the same way. Remember always, that the left hemisphere of the brain and the right side of the body are electrical, the right hemisphere of the brain and the left side of the body are magnetic, and give your treatments accordingly, and you will find you will be able to apply the Sex principle in healing, in the most perfect and most efficacious manner conceivable.

It should be borne in mind that the sunlight is electrical and the moonlight, magnetic, consequently sun baths may be found very efficacious for patients who need more masculinity, more of the electrical force, but should never be indulged in by persons who have too much, and require magnetism or feminine force. Moonlight walks at night, sleeping in a room where the moonlight can enter, getting in connection with moonlight, will be valuable for those needing more magnetism or feminine influence. For this reason it will be found that ordinarily it is better for women to take sun baths and men moon baths, only in cases where women are suffering from sexual impotency, when moonlight is very desirable for them, and in cases of sexual weakness in men, sunlight will be found advantageous. For the same reason, it is found that women ordinarily prefer hot baths, and hot baths are better for them because they draw off the magnetism of the women and impart the electrical force, and so, in a limited degree, will be found to be on the same principle as a love affair; while cold baths are much better for men, drawing off the superabundance of electrical force and imparting more magnetism, and will be found quite as valuable as a liaison. However, there is an exception to this in cases of men who are sexually weak, who want to become more masculine. Such men should bathe in warm water; and women who require more femininity should bathe in cold water, as in this way they will draw off some of the masculinity and take on more of the feminine or magnetic principle. Any application of this general rule will be found to be an application of the general law of Sexual Healing.

Sexual Healing is simply the application to therapeutic uses, of this principle of sex polarity, which is found to work throughout all nature.

METAPHYSICAL HEALING

These lessons are the practical experience of Metaphysics applied to disease in all its aspects to restore Health on all planes, Physical, Astral, Mental, Soul and Spirit. They show how to master disease and gain and retain what the world is seeking, Equilibrium and Health

By
DR. A. S. RALEIGH

Volume II

A Course of Private Lessons given
to his personal pupils

THE HERMETIC PUBLISHING COMPANY

3006 Lake Park Ave.   Chicago, Ill., U. S. A.

CONTENTS

L E S S O N

on

P H R E N O - T H E R A P E U T I C S

In the early days when Phrenology was developing to the point of an exact science, in 1832, to 1835, along there and in the years following, the study of Animal Magnetism attracted considerable attention and Professor O. S. Fowler, at that time came to the conclusion that the Phrene Organs of the Brain and the mind were really the mental poles of the diverse parts of the body and that by the stimulation of those organs it would be possible to develop the different parts of the body and to strengthen their activity. In other words, that functional diseases of the body could be cured by applying magnetism to their phrene organs and in this way strengthening them. The organ, or muscle, in a word, could be stimulated, not by applying magnetism to it direct, but by applying it to its phrene organ.

This was Fowler's theory which, however, he was not able to verify by experiment. In the course of time Fowler passed away without having tried this theory. We discovered, by accident, the truth of the general principle, and in a number of experiments worked it out, demonstrating it to be correct. We know at the present time that every organ of the body, every muscle, every nerve center, has its corresponding pole in the brain; not only that, but every brain center has a corresponding pole in the body or the face, the hands, the feet, or wherever it may be.

The system of Phreno-Therapeutics which we have developed, consists of the application of magnetism to the Phrene Organs which govern those functional organs of the body. Consequently, if a man's body is out of order we should find out what the trouble is and find the phrene organ which governs that organ of the body, which controls and regulates that function and by the application of magnetism or some other method of stimulation, we will be able to direct a current of energy to that organ to build it up, strengthen it and give it new force.

The first organ we want to consider is ALIMENTIVENESS, lying just forward from the ear and back of the Temple. This is the lowest organ in the head, forward from the ear, that is rather on the side of the head, coming down to the face. The front of the Organ is really the Organ of Bibativeness, giving the desire for liquids, and back of this the desire for solids. Now, as a matter of fact, this organ of Alimentiveness, including Bibativeness, is the pole of the stomach and the entire digestive tract and regulates the digestive process. It is the Center of Appetite and also gives the power for satisfying that appetite. It is in two divisions, Bibativeness regulating the assimilation of liquids of all kinds—water, soups, milk, coffee, tea, wine, whisky,— everything in the liquid form, in fact, is included under the head of Bibativeness, while all solid foods are included under the head of Alimentiveness. If the stomach is weak this organ will be found to be correspondingly weak. If on the other hand, the stomach is strong, able to digest anything, this organ will be found to be very strong and vice versa. As the body develops through the strengthening of the digestive processes, this organ will be found to develop and as this organ develops so the strength of the stomach and the digestive processes will develop also. The secretion of gastric juice, or pepsin, of the pancreatic juice and everything of that kind, all the digestive fluids, in fact, is governed by this organ. Likewise, also the secretion of saliva, the glands in the mouth which secrete saliva are also governed in this way by this organ. It is the function of this organ, in other words, to supply stimulus to all of those special organs which operate in that way.

The time will come when, as a result of the study of Psycho- physiological sarcology, there will be discovered in this organ, an organ governing each of those physical organs. It will be found to be not only a faculty, but a group of more than a dozen distinct faculties, but at the present time we know it as only one faculty although we know that it governs all those functions, sending the stimuli to the diverse organs, and thus enabling them to perform their functions.

If there is found in a patient, difficulty in digesting solid food, he can live on liquids all right, then that part of the organ ordinarily called Alimentiveness, lying nearest the ear, should be strengthened, and the way to do this is to stand back of your patient's chair, then place your fingers of the right hand over the organ on the right side of the head and the fingers of the left hand over the organs on the left side of the head so that your hands will become a battery, the positive pole being placed on the right side, which is the negative pole of the brain, and the negative hand on the left side, which is the positive pole, thus establishing the complete connection. Then, by a process of treatment, transmit the healing force from your body into the brain of your patient, let the treatment last fifteen or twenty minutes, if need be, continually keeping a stream of energy flowing into that brain, stimulating it, building it up, and at the same time fixing your consciousness upon the digestive processes, picturing the changes which you wish to take place, seeing them as already taking place. Never tell it to do so by and by, but always direct it right now.

It should be borne in mind also that a lack of appetite, loss of appetite is due to the inability of the system to adapt itself to the use of food, therefore, if the appetite be poor and you want to restore it, simply go to work and treat the the organ in the same way.

Bibativeness, when weak causes inability to digest liquid food, and should be treated for this purpose, building it up in order to give ability to handle liquid foods.

If, on the other hand, you find the difficulty manifests itself by a lack of appetite rather than inability to handle food, treat it just the same, to build up and restore the appetite. If you find there is a strong appetite for liquids, too much, too strong, as is manifested in the toper, then the desire for food should be stimulated in the place of the desire for liquids.

People who are corpulent are so largely because of too great an activity of the faculty of Bibativeness, because they get food from the use of liquids, to a great extent. Also this organ of Bibativeness gives capacity for absorption to a much greater degree than is found in other persons. People with a large development of this faculty not only handle liquids, but also absorb a great deal of liquids. There are persons who drink as much as two gallons of water daily and absorb the larger quantity of it. Others cannot handle it at all. We have seen people who could not drink more than a pint of water a day. The ability to consume large quantities of liquids consists of the ability to absorb them and this capacity for absorption is the cause of the putting on of adipose tissue.

Patients who are too corpulent should be restrained from consuming so much liquid, so that they will not absorb so much and in such cases the faculty of Alimentiveness should be developed to a certain extent and not the faculty of Bibativeness. On the contrary if a patient is too thin, if he needs to put on tissue, develop the faculty of Bibativeness, giving increased power of absorption and in this way he will improve greatly in health.

Vitativeness, the organ lying back of the middle of the ear, gives desire of life and is, therefore the organ to be stimulated in treatment of melancholia when it manifests itself in the form of disinterestedness in life, and indifference to life. This may be overcome by stimulating that faculty so as to bring about a greater desire for life. Not only so, but this organ gives vitality. It is the center in which is developed that vitative power, vital energy, or Prana, in other words. There are a great many forms of energy produced in the system. They are all manifestations of one form, but there are organs provided in the brain for the purpose of preparing special forms of energy to be employed in carrying on the work of the system. Not only is this true, but there also are organs of the body adapted to the work of preparing those forces so that they may be adapted to physical uses. The preparation of vital energy is the function of Vitativeness and a low state of vitality may be remedied by the application of magnetism or psychical force to this organ in the same general way as would be done in treating Alimentiveness.

Just below this organ is the organ of Amativeness, lying at the base of the brain, reaching from back of the lower part of the ears clear around to the back of the brain. This, however, is divided into two organs, two subdivisions. That part on the side of the head, back of the ears gives the love of sex as it ordinarily expresses itself, and might be ordinarily termed masculinity and femininity as it may occur in man or woman, giving a more positive or a more negative character to the being, and if this be wanting in a person, if he be weakly sexed, and the sex needs strengthening, of course, it should be done by the application of Magnetism to this part of the brain.

That part lying at the back of the head, the extreme base of the brain, is the organ of Reproduction, which gives the instinct for reproduction, the desire for offspring and for cohabitation. At the same time it gives virility. It gives the power of reproduction, and all forms of sexual impotency be they in either man or woman, are due to an extreme weakness of this part of the brain. Such complaints should be treated, therefore, by an application of magnetism to this part of the brain, it being the pole which governs the sexual organ and it is because of this fact that the treatment of sexual weakness has been so terribly futile. Physicicans undertake to treat the organs locally when, as a matter of fact, it is not a local trouble at all; it is a lack of sexual force, because the sex energy for the purpose of reproduction, is manufactured, generated here in this part of the brain, and the sexual organs cannot perform their functions without the energy through which such functions are to be performed. This energy, we say, is produced here, therefore, this part of the brain should be stimulated in order that it may acquire the ability to generate this force. The sex energy which is not used on the physical plane, that which is manifested on the higher planes is generated in that part of the organ denominated the Love of Sex, and if it be found weak in this respect, must be stimulated here.

The power for executing anything which may be in the mind, the power for applying one's executiveness, in other words, lies in a development of the organ of Destructiveness, the front part of this organ, lying a little forward of the middle of the ear, but up over the ear, just back of Alimentiveness, and the ability to work, to carry out something, is found in the organ of work which is the rear half of the organ, coming downward over the ear, down to Vitativeness. Inability to carry out work, which a great many people consider to be chronic,

10

laziness and an evidence of total depravity, is in reality nothing but an undeveloped, languid or dormant state of this part of the brain, and by the application of Magnetism, the stimulation of this faculty, all indisposition to work, languor and indifference to things will disappear.

The Organ of Agreeableness, lying downward on either side of Human Nature toward the side of the head is in two divisions, Blandness, which is toward the top, and Youthfulness, a little lower down. It has been a problem among phrenologists to find why this Organ of Agreeableness should be associated with Youthfulness, why it should give the youthful character, etc., but as a matter of fact it not only does that, but it prevents old age, it prevents the ageing process. One who is agreeable, one who is trying to please, to make people happy, in a way to be entertaining, is developing a tendency which rouses the youthful vibration in his being and will prevent the ageing process. To apply magnetism to the upper part of this Organ would simply develop Blandness. It is the lower part which gives the youthful character and the sprightly agreeable tendencies manifested in youth, and these activities will, as a matter of fact, have the effect of rejuvenating the entire body, and will make it younger.

The Organ of Tone, lying backward from Time and below Mirthfulness and forward from Constructiveness, is in two divisions, namely, Melody and Harmony. The latter lying backward from Melody. This organ of Harmony gives, of course, an appreciation of Harmony. It is from this that the musician gets his harmony, and it is not simply this, but it also develops a state of harmony, harmony of vibration throughout the entire system from head to feet. The vibrations and circulations of the system are carried on in strict accordance with harmony. Discord is eliminated from the system and harmony is established as a result of the activity of this organ. Harmony being the keynote of health, being the influence which is most promotive of health, health, in fact, being nothing but a state of harmony, the development and stimulation of this organ will conduce unto a state of harmony and therefore of health. The greatest healing force for the body is, therefore, the harmony which will emanate from the activity of this organ.

Application, lying back of Continuity, is the extreme back of the head, and just below Self-Esteem, gives not only the tendency, the desire to applying one's self to anything, but gives the power, the "stick-to-it-ive-ness" in other words, which will keep one from wandering from one thing to another. The inability to stay with a certain thing is not, therefore, a physical defect in the ordinary sense, but a mental defect and must be treated by the application of magnetism to that part of the brain.

Color blindness in any degree, is due to a weakness of the Organ of Color, lying just below the eye, and just backward from the sight. The strength of that organ is manifested by the elevation of the eyebrows at that particular point; its weakness is indicated by a depression of that part of the eye. The more highly developed this organ is the more acute will be one's sense of color, one's ability to differentiate between shades and tints, while one who is weak in this organ will scarcely recognize the secondary colors. Our father, for instance, never was able to tell any difference between blue and green. Color blindness is, therefore, due simply to an undeveloped or dormant state of this faculty and can in every case be removed by the quickening and development of the faculty, that is by the application of magnetism, in the same way we would treat the other faculties.

Now the faculty of Order, lies just outward, just back of Color and manifests itself first in Neatness and then a little further back in System. It may not occur to the average person as being a disease when he is wanting in order, wanting in neatness or system, but we consider one of the most serious diseases to which the human family is subject, to be want of order and system and in the conduct of affairs. If a person is not neat or not systematic in his way of carrying on things, this Organ should be developed, and it should also be borne in mind that this Organ of System, if it be extremely weak is liable to affect the physiological condition, so that the different functions of the body do not act in Harmony; a person gets so that everything is chaotic in his actions, so he will be chaotic in his manner of life in what he does, and everything of the kind, in his very functional activities. In order that the system may be clean it is also necessary that this faculty of Neatness should be extremely active, for the faculty not only gives the desire for neatness, the tendency for neatness, but the diverse parts of the body also respond. Unless this faculty is, therefore, sufficiently strong it will not keep the system clean. Disease of either type, that is where there is no system, where the body is chaotic, or where it is filthy and is not sufficiently purging out the impurities, should in either case be treated by a proper development of the proper part of the organ.

A weakness of the Organ of Weight, which lies forward from Color, just above the sight of the eye, manifests itself in difficulty in preserving the center of gravity. A man who cannot stand up on his feet, so to speak, who cannot stand on level ground, has this difficulty because of a weakness of the Organ of Weight. He cannot preserve his equilibrium and thus his whole system is thrown out of order. For a difficulty of this kind, a difficulty which we ordinarily attribute to a lack of steadiness, of nerve, we should develop the Organ of Weight by the application of Magnetism to it, and when it is developed we will find the difficulty in maintaining the center of gravity will immediately pass away.

One of the most important organs is that of Physical Observation, which manifests itself in a prominence just above the bridge of the nose, running in fact, from the bridge of the nose up between the eyebrows and a little above, manifesting itself in a prominence there and also an elevation. Now, this is really the center of all physical senses, seeing, hearing, tasting, smelling, touching, and everything of the kind; they all have their center in this organ, and so if there be weakness in any of those senses, in the auditory, olfactory, gustatory, or tactile nerves as the case may be, apply magnetism to that part of the brain and you find those nerves will become more sensitive, and practically all those defects will be removed. Not only that, but a weakness in the accommodating muscles of the eye, or any of the other organs may be cured in the same way.

We should bear in mind, however, that there are a number of facial poles which may be employed the same as those in the head. It is almost as important to treat the facial poles properly as those in the cranium.

Between the corners of the mouth and the ears we have situated the pole of digestion. It may also be used in treating the stomach. Between that and the corner of the mouth, right back over the hectic flush which first comes in the case of consumption, is the facial pole of the lungs and by the stimulation of that with magnetism, the lungs may be cured, and any case of consumption can be cured if stimuli be applied there in time.

In the lip, right in the front part of the lip, right in the center, is the pole of Amativeness. It is for this reason that during the courting season man and woman always kiss with that part of the mouth; you never see them kiss any other way. Amativeness naturally expresses itself there and is indicated by a prominence and thickness of that part of the lip, but remember it is at the edge of the lip, the termination of the lip and stimulation of that part will consequently give strength to the reproductive power, or the amorous power, in a way, not so much the reproductive power as the love of sex.

Now, right in the corner of the mouth, but still on the upper lip is the pole of Parental Love and a prominence of that part of the mouth or lip will give the power for procreation, for parentage, while midway between the corner and the center of the lip a prominence indicates Platonic love, fraternity, etc.

Now, in the lip and above the edge, between that and the nose is the Will. The longer the lip is, therefore, the more powerful is the force of Will. This is what is meant by the admonition to "Keep a stiff upper lip." By the development of that, that is by the application of Magnetism, it will be found that the power of the Will will be strengthened.

In weak eyes we find that the eyeball gradually sinks, consequently in a case of this kind Magnetism should be applied in order to bring it out.

Generally speaking the upper part of the head, from the eyes upward, indicate the intellect, from the mouth upward the emotions, and downward the physical powers, though this is not always the case, and by stimulation of those parts of the body we may stimulate the organs which they represent and consequently the parts of the body which are under their control.

There is a statement in the Bible that Joy doeth good like a medicine, and sorrow drieth up the bones and in this sense it is true and the Organ of Hope and also the Organ of Mirthfulness will be found exercising a very great healing influence when stimulated, by reason of the vitalizing essences which they pour forth.

If you wish to treat a certain local trouble in this way and do not know its phrene organ, it will ordinarily be found sufficient to press the hands closely on the head; go over the head completely with considerable percussion with the fingers. The moment you feel a sensation in the organ which you want to treat — remember you should go over your own head and when you feel in that organ the sensation, or in fact, any sensation, know that you have found the mental pole, the cranial pole of that organ located the same place on the head of your patient; apply magnetism there and you will succeed in reaching the organ and thus strengthening it.

In the treatment of functional diseases it will be found that this Phreno-Therapeutic method is more than ten times as efficacious as the application of magnetism direct to the bodily organ could be, because you are now touching the center, as it were, the spring which directs the current and which is supplying the power to that organ. You are at the same time developing it so that it will of its own volition as it were, produce much more power than it did previously.

This is, in brief, the system. It may be applied in almost any way. It is simply the application of the magnetic or psychical force to the phrene organs, governing the different functional centers of the body and as you apply this force, quickening and stimulating an organ, and therefore, sending forth a current of energy, charging, vitalizing, magnetizing the organ which is weak, you will thus build it up, strengthen it, compel it to perform its function. It is the natural method of stimulating the diverse organs of the body, and will be found to be effective in every instance no matter what the trouble may be.

L E S S O N
O N
P S Y C H I C A L   H E A L I N G

The main difference between Psychical and Magnetic Healing is that whereas the magnetic force which is used in Magnetic Healing is generated in the organs of Vitativeness and Amativeness, being what we might term Vital Magnetism and also being closely allied to the Sexual Force, — in fact, being Sexual Force in a slightly different form and when generated solely through amativeness, being that force absolutely.

In Psychical Healing we employ the Psychical Force which is generated in the Organ of Spirituality. This force being generated there, may be used for the healing of the body. Inasmuch as it possesses a much higher rate of vibration, being not Physical or Astral, but of a Soul Character, it is of much more force for healing purposes than the ordinary magnetism or anything of that kind. Because of its higher rate of vibration, it is able to raise the Aura so far above the plane of disease that those discordant conditions will become impossible.

There are two ways in which this healing force may be employed. The first is to stimulate the activity of the organ of Spirituality so that it will generate a much greater quantity of psychical force than ordinarily, at the same time directing this force to the part of the body where it is needed.

The other method is to transmit the psychical Force from the organism of the Healer into that of the patient.

In the first method there are also two divisions. The first is by Suggestion, to stimulate that faculty. This is performed by making such statements or motions or anything else, whatever it may be, as will stimulate the organ by reason of calling up those pictures in mind, suggesting to the imagination or thought or emotions, those things of a spiritual character, so that in this way, the organ will be made to act.

The other method is by the application of magnetism or psychical force to that part of the brain so that it will, in this objective manner so to speak, be stimulated.

To follow the latter practice, the Healer should have the patient seated in a chair and stand behind the chair. He should then place the Electrical Hand on the Magnetic Faculty; that is to say, the right hand should be placed on the right side of the head and the left hand on the left side, so that the electrical hand will be over the Magnetic Faculty and the Magnetic Hand over the Electrical Faculty, and then, by concentration, of the mind, send the energy down through the right hand, into the Magnetic Faculty, then letting it pass out across and from the Magnetic Faculty, through the Electrical Faculty back into the hand, so that the circuit will be closed, passing through the hand to and through the brain of the patient back to the hand again.

Now, in this way, having the circuit closed, concentrate the mind and drive the force, the psychical force, from the body into the brain of the patient.

Inasmuch as it is the natural function of the organ of Spirituality to generate Psychical Force, as well as a number of other things, it is also its natural function to receive the spiritual force from above, consequently when negatively polarized, it is able to receive the psychical force with the greatest freedom.

In this way you can practice either the method of transmitting the force or you can stimulaate the faculty. It makes no difference which it is. This is the best method to pursue.

Of course, if you want to simply stimulate the faculty, you should transmit the force to the organ of Spirituality. It makes no difference about what becomes of it afterwards; you simply transmit the force there and then keep your mind concentrated upon the idea of stimulating that faculty, and while in this concentration, the hands on the head, you should form in mind a picture of the awakening of the faculty, see it awakened, becoming more active, being stimulated into new life, new activity. It is a very good idea to have some definite thought in your mind which will stimulate this picture and while you continue to hold the hands there maintain an attitude of positive concentration, always affirming the awakening of the faculty. It is being quickened, stimulated, aroused, excited, etc., in such a way as to call out all the energy that there is in it; it is generating more energy, etc. Everything which has the tendency of awakening and stimulating the faculty, filling it with new life and energy, putting it to work, will be found effective, as the one all-important thing for you to realize in this work is the activity of the faculty. That is what you want to demand if you can bring about that condition it will generate a sufficient quantity of the psychical force.

But if you want to follow the other method you must, by concentration of mind, transmit to this faculty the requisite quantity of psychical force continually driving it in. Then the picture, in addition to being one of the awakening, quickening and stimulation of the faculty, must also be one which will represent the flowing in of the psychical force from your body, through your fingers, into the Faculty of Spirituality. You must see streams of this energy flowing in, through the organ of spirituality into the body of the patient. Let the currents flow in. As you see this in your mind's eye, as you imagine the inflowing currents of force, they will actually flow in, for it is by the imagination, by the concentration of the mind that the force is directed and as you direct it in this way, so will it go.

By this concentration of mind, you will be able to transmit the psychical force to the organism of your patient; that is to say, you will get it in there and at the same time you will be awakening the organ of Spirituality, because as it passes through that organ it must necessarily quicken that and make it work and thus it will generate more spiritual force or psychical force at the same time it is receiving that from you. For this reason Psychical Healing is far more efficacious than Magnetic Healing.

Another thing, you do not have to place your hands anywhere else. The psychical force being of a higher order than magnetism, will much more easily respond to the direction of the consciousness than the magnetic force; in fact, it is of a higher order than mind itself, being really on the Buddhic Plane. The concentration, therefore, must be of a very high quality; merely intellectual or emotional concentration will not direct it. You may simply fix your attention on that part of the body where you want to direct it and it will immediately go there, or you may mark out the path which you wish it to travel, the nerves over which it must travel, or nerve center it has to reach, and it will follow your intelligent direction, traveling over those nerves and charging, magnetizing that nerve center or plexus, ganglion or whatever it may be. If you do not know this you may simply concentrate on that organ or muscle, that part of the body you want it to go to and when you concentrate there, your attention will carry the psychical force directly there so that it will permeate that part of the body, will fill it with new vitality, build it up and strengthen it.

You may thus concentrate upon the hand or arm, the foot, the lungs, whatever it may be and while fixing the attention there, at the same time continually transmitting a stream of psychical force into the body, you will carry it to that part of the body. This should be distinctly borne in mind. You do not merely diffuse the force through the body, but if you keep the attention fixed on a definite part of the body all that you put in through the organ of spirituality will go there. The only way to diffuse it through the body is to fix your attention that way, let your attention go through the body from head to feet, and whatever you suggest for it to do when it is going that way, it will do. It absolutely responds to the attention which you give to the body. For instance, if you direct it to eliminate certain poisons from the body, it will spend itself in this way. If you direct it to build

17

up new tissue, it will do so. If you direct it to give strength, vitality, energy to that part of the body, it will do so. If you direct it to heal up a wound, it will do so. In a word, the psychical force has the power of performing any function appertaining to the human organism, no matter what it may be. It is in deed and in truth a "Cure-all." There is no disease to which flesh is heir but what it will cure, and it will cure one just as easily as it will another. The work which it performs depends upon what you tell it to perform.

Remember then, that the universal medicine is being placed in the body of the patient, by your treatment and you are thus giving to his body a force which is capable of doing anything imaginable. By fixing of your attention on a definite part of the body, a defnite organ or nerve center, whatever it may be, you are directing that force to a given point so that all that you put in the body is sent to that point.

Likewise, by fixing your attention on what you want it to do, by concentrating the mind in such a way as to form a clear picture of the work which it has to do, you will cause it to perform any function that you may have in mind. Remember, however, that in giving this direction, you are not to tell it to do this after a while, not to have the idea that it should later on do so and so, but you are to direct it to do it now, for it is only while that picture is held in your mind that the energy is being so directed. It is the picture held in mind that directs the activity of this force, therefore, you should, in your consciousness, see it performing certain functions here and now. Give your positive directions continually, maintaining in mind the picture of the work, so that it will go ahead and perform it. Always bear in mind that the workman is the Psychical Force, but the foreman who directs this force and directs its labor, is the picture which is in the mind of the Healer. The danger is if you do not do this, you will leave an undirected force in the system which will respond to the pictures you form. Consequently afterwards if you form a picture there without reference to its therapeutic value, your suggestion giving direction to the picture, which you might not wish to form in the mind of your patient, nevertheless, it will direct the activity of this force and thus you may accomplish results which would not be at all desirable. Likewise, if you leave an unemployed force in the body of the patient, he, himself may form mental pictures which will direct the operation of this force and will accomplish very undesirable results.

The whole key to Psychical Healing is, briefly, to impart the psychical force from your own organism, through the organ of Spirituality of the patient into his body. The more you put in there, the better, and this is accomplished by concentration of the mind positively and by maintaining the concentration and all the attention on

18

the Soul Plane, by maintaining the activity of your own Organ of Spirituality and thus transmitting the force to the body of the patient.

Second: Transmitting this force to a given part of the body by the fixing of the attention upon that point and keeping it there through the entire treatment.

Third: By maintaining in the consciousness a picture of the result which you wish to accomplish as being actually enacted before you.

Lastly: In never leaving any of the Psychical Force within the patient which has not been directed and employed.

If you will observe these directions you will find no difficulty in the world in perfectly employing this wonderful healing method and in curing all the ills to which flesh is heir by the mere application of the psychical force.

It should be borne in mind also that this method is far more safely employed than the magnetic method because this being a soul force and not a physical or an astral force, is not influenced by the condition of the body as the magnetism is. For instance there is no danger of ever transmitting a diseased condition which exists in the healer, through Psychical Healing, and this is almost certain to take place in Magnetic Healing. Also, the condition of the passions will never effect the psychical force while they do in Magnetic Healing. Even the mental states, beliefs, etc. will not effect the patient as they would in Magnetic Healing.

None of those undesirable conditions can possibly take place because it is no part of the physical, mental or astral being of the healer, therefore, can never have any effect of that kind. Neither will it influence those principles except as it raised their vibrations.

At the same time it should be borne in mind that this method will make the patient more spiritual, will develop the soul quality within himself, and the psychical healer is a physician of souls as well as bodies.

For one who is able to perform this kind of healing, it therefore, becomes decidedly desirable that it should be made use of in preference to all other methods with the single exception of Spiritual or Divine Healing. But in order to do this the mind and soul of the healer must be kept from the lower elements. The passions must not be allowed to operate, in fact, the healer must function upon the Buddhic Plane while he is giving the treatments, his whole consciousness must be fixed in the realm of soul, otherwise he will not transmit soul force but magnetism.

He must keep his consciousness fixed there and thus be in a state of Cosmic Consciousness. If he is not, it will be impossible for him to transmit the psychical force.

It will also be borne in mind that it will depend upon the spirituality of the healer generally, to the degree to which he can enter into this condition which is necessary to give the right kind of psychical treatments. The more spiritual a person is, the more thoroughly he is identified with the Buddhic Plane, the greater skill he will have in this kind of work.

The size and activity of the organ of spirituality will, therefore, determine the ability of a person to perform Psychical Healing. Let it be distinctly understood here and now that no person with small spirituality can learn to practice Psychical Healing. The Psychical Healing requires absolutely a high development of spirituality. The larger that organ is and the more active it is, the greater will be his healing power no matter whether he knows anything about the scientific application of it or not. The technical knowledge of Psychical Healing is one thing, but the power to heal is another thing. One who has large spirituality and who is positive so that he is able to transmit it and who has the power of concentration, whether he knows anything at all about the method, can do more than ten times as much as one who has a perfect understanding of the system, but who has a small development of spirituality.

Now, spirituality makes one naturally religious. We do not mean by this that he believes any particular religious creed or anything of that kind, but we do mean that he is naturally religious, that he is what many would term superstitious, one who has faith. By religion in this respect, we do not mean worship, but we mean faith, we mean that he believes in God; he knows — that God and the Divine are true. To the spiritual man the super-natural is much more real than the natural. Such a man can do this kind of healing, no other man can. It is utterly useless for a rationalist, one who believes in nature only and denies the supernatural, to try to perform Psychical Healing. No matter how much he knows about those things he has not the power to do it; he hasn't the healing force unless that healing force is generated in his organ of spirituality, and if that organ is small, of course, it is unable to generate very much of this force.

This is really the secret of the healing saints who have been found in all religions. They have had faith and by reason of their faith they have had great spirituality, great soul force and that force has been transmitted to the bodies of their patients. In other words they have had big souls and, by reason of their largeness of soul they have been able to exercise healing power.

Now, there is no use for the little souls to undertake to duplicate their work. They have simply been overflowing with the psychical power and wherever they have fixed their attention they have directed it. This is the secret of the natural healer, who does those wonderful works of healing. Magnetic healing cannot duplicate it. It is possible only by reason of the great psychical force which is overflowing the very being of their healer.

The great mistake which so many of the healing systems of the present day make, is in assuming that it is merely the mind. They can see nothing higher than the mind. They say that if there is any soul beyond the mind they do not know what it is, while as a matter of fact the healing power is found to increase in direct ratio to the spirituality, unselfishness, purity, morality and saintliness of character of the healer and to decrease in direct ratio to his immorality, impurity and selfishness without reference to his intellectual power.

The healing power, therefore, does not depend upon intellect, it does not depend upon the power of concentration, it does not depend upon the imagination. These are simply means of directing the power, they are very important because without them, the force will not be properly directed, but will be scattered and thus will not be employed to the best advantage. But the power itself, consists of spirituality. The more spiritual a person is, the more power he possesses, consequently the person who would be an effective psychical healer must first develop his organ of Spirituality.

Second: He must live on the Buddhic Plane as much of the time as possible and try to the best of his ability to entirely identify himself with it.

Third: He must renounce everything which will in any way interfere with his spirituality.

Fourth: He must develop the power of concentration to the highest possible point.

Fifth: He must learn to fix the attention on a given point and

Sixth: He must develop a vivid imagination which will enable him to see the mental pictures necessary for carrying on the work.

Seventh: It will be found necessary for him to become as positive as possible.

Eighth: He must use this psychical force which this will develop, for healing purposes, not for other purposes. For instance, one cannot be a great teacher and a great healer both, if he does very much of either one. The psychical force is developed, but it naturally follows those channels which it has acquired the habit of following. The teacher, therefore, will naturally use up his psychical force in teaching; the writer in his writing; whatever it may be that he does, it will naturally follow that channel. The healer, therefore, must follow healing to the exclusion of everything else if he would reach the highest attainments along this line. Thus he will be enabled to accomplish a great deal.

The healer must be sure that he does not do anything, keep up any practice which will interfere with the development of his spirituality. That is the all-important point to be borne in mind. It is for this reason that healers of this type have usually maintained the position that it was better not to charge anything for their healing, to give the treatments free of charge, than to charge money, the reason being that if they charged money for it and followed it as a business it was liable to develop their selfishness. They were not likely to have the interest of the patient at heart sufficiently, but would rather give way to those thoughts which would call up the lower principles and take them down from the Buddhic Plane and consequently they would not transmit the psychical force but magnetism. This, however, does not necessarily follow from charging a fee, if the fee be reasonable, if the healer has the interest of the patient at heart and his healing is not for his own interest so much as for the good of the patient and he at the same time realizes that he must have a compensation; he must live in order to do this. If his fee is a means to an end, namely the means of enabling him to do more work of this kind, accomplish more good, then this difficulty will not arise. If he also realizes that it is necessary to make charges in order to accomplish the best results it will be found absolutely necessary that he will do what will ac-complish the most good, consequently in charging the patient a mod-erate fee he is really making the patient appreciate the value of the treatment and consequently doing the patient good. For this reason the acceptance of a fee will not in any way interfere with that perfect unselfishness, that Buddhic consciousness which is essential unto the perfect accomplishment of the work and in this way he will be able to transmit the healing force because he will maintain his consciousness upon that plane of perfect unselfishness and thus he will be generating the spiritual or soul force and transmitting it to his patient and thus will accomplish the best possible results.

Remember, however, that the one point to be borne in mind is that Spirituality gives the psychical force that is used in Psychical Heal-ing. The other methods are merely methods of direction applied to that force. The concentration, the fixing of the attention, the mental pic-ture even the placing of the hands and everything of that kind are merely so many details to be employed in the healing of the patient, so many details employed for the direction of the healing force which is generated in the organ of Spirituality and which, therefore, can only be governed by reason of the Spirituality of the healer.

L E S S O N
O N
S P I R I T U A L   H E A L I N G

The only difference between Spiritual Healing and Psychical
Healing is, that whereas in Psychical Healing the force that is employed is psychical force generated within the Organ of Spirituality
in the Healer, that is to say, he is using his own psychical force, is
transmitting this through the Organ of Spirituality in his patient to
the different parts of the body and thus accomplishing the healing,—
whereas, in Spiritual Healing or Divine Healing he is not using his
own force, but is using the Spirit of God to accomplish the work. The
method is precisely the same. You stand back of your patient and
place the right hand on the right side of the head, the left hand on
the left side, placing the fingers over the Organ of Spirituality.
Then you begin your treatment in the same way you would in psychical
healing, transmitting the current down to the hand and into the brain,
through his Organ of Spirituality, and from there over the system,
directing it wherever you will, simply by fixing the attention upon
that part of the body where you want the current to go and as long as
you keep the attention concentrated upon any given point you are maintaining the current of force there in that particular part of the body.
Or, you may sweep a current through the body from head to foot, stimulating all the cells and tissues, nerves, etc., in the body to action.
In this way the current may be able to have a general influence upon the
body from head to foot, or in case you want to drive out some disease,
something like scrofula or eczema, you want to make it come to the
surface, you simply cause the force to go through and through the body
and then by concentration of the attention, cause it to flow out from
the center of the body to the surface, until finally it flows out through
the pores of the skin. In this way you can bring this diseased tissue
to the surface and ultimately cure anything in that way. You can carry
out effete matter and all the poisons that may be accumulated in the
system.

The cure of poisoning may be accomplished in this way or you can change the vibration of the body, the Aura and everything by simply causing it to flow through the entire system, and then to keep in mind this vibration, holding it in relation to the vibratory forces of the body until they are raised up, brought into this state of vibratory harmony. It should be borne in mind, however, that it is not your psychical force you are using when you are performing spiritual healing. Spiritual Healing is another force, in fact, it is the Spirit of God in the highest aspect.

Of course, there are two kinds of Spiritual Healing. Spiritual Healing in the strictest sense of the word is not the Spirit of God, but the Universal Spirit, that is drawn into the being by elevating the individual spirit until it unites for the time being, with the Universal Spirit.

A person to do this kind of healing must be a Para-Nirvani, or at least he must be functioning on the plane of Para-Nirvana at the time he is giving the treatment in order that he may be filled with an influx of that Universal Spirit and thus his Organ of Spirituality becomes the channel through which that spiritual force pours into his system. It streams in there and fills his system through and through until his whole being is charged with it. He becomes a magnet and is thus able to transmute this healing spiritual force to the organism of the patient.

Now, this kind of healing is not magnetic healing, neither is it psychical healing. The force is of a higher order, instituting a much higher vibration, and will accomplish all the work that the other healing methods accomplish with none of the other evil consequences. But it is possible to do this only when you can lose sight of your personality, your individuality; as long as he contemplates himself as being separate and apart, it is utterly impossible for him to accomplish this phase of healing. It is necessary for a person in order to accomplish Spiritual Healing, to thoroughly identify himself with the Universal Spirit and at the same time to have his patient identified in his consciousness with this Universal Spirit, so that there is no difference. His spirit and that of his patient are identical and they are in turn, identical with the Universal Spirit, consequently he is simply a channel through which that Universal Spirit flows, and thus his Organ of Spirituality is the medium by which Brahman is able to flow in; becomes the channel through which it flows in through his hands, into the Organ of Spirituality of his patient, and thus through his entire body.

A spiritual healer then must be the medium, the modulating chord, as it were, between the patient and the Universal Spirit, and his capacity to heal depends upon his ability to accomplish this work, to become in deed and in truth, the modulating chord which will bring harmony between his patient and the Universal Spirit.

24

Now, it should be borne in mind that spiritual healing is through the Spirit, not through the body, that is to say you must bring your patient's spirit into union with the Universal Spirit and thus his spirit is first awakened, spiritualized, filled with the Universal Spirit. The union has been accomplished so far as the spirit is concerned. Then this must flow in until the soul is awakened and filled with the spirit, — brought into union and harmony, then down to the Causal Body, the Mental Body, the Astral Body, Etheric Double, until at last the gross Physical Body is brought into union. The Universal Spirit now reigns supreme throughout the entire being of the patient. It is in this way that Spiritual Healing is accomplished.

What really is the cause of sickness and weakness, and everything of that kind? Is it not because of individualism? Is it not because the patient has separated from the universe, is no longer a part of the Kosmos, but has separated himself as it were, and thus is starving for the want of this spiritual force? Now, the healer becomes the modulating chord through which the patient is brought back into harmony, his entire being is made to perfectly harmonize with the universal spirit, and thus that spirit is enabled to come forth into manifestation, to manifest itself in and through his entire being. When you realize this, you will understand why it is that the Spiritual Healer must be one who is in perfect harmony, for the time being with the Universal Spirit. But this is not all, — he must also be in harmony with his patient. He must be able to sympathize with the patient, to enter into rapport with him and thus act as the medium between the Universal Spirit and the Individual Spirit. It is for this reason that those who have performed this kind of healing have usually adopted the rule of charging no money for what they do. They do the work gratuitously because that will enable them to be in a more sympathetic state in relation to the patient, than they could be ordinarily, if they charged money for it. They sympathize more with those they are serving, to whom they are giving something, than they would likely to with persons who were paying them money for what they did. However, one who has the proper degree of sympathy and who charges money, not in the sense of payment for what he is doing, but to enable him to live so that he may be able to do more good — his reception of money under these conditions would not be detrimental. But remember, it is sympathy that establishes the connection between the Healer and the Patient, so that he is able to transmit the healing spirit, and it is self-forgetfulness, self-abnegation, that establishes the harmony between the healer and the Universal Spirit.

Remember then, that the healer is merely the channel through which the Universal Spirit flows into the patient, he is a mediator, a condenser, as it were, one who brings about the state of connection between the spirit and the individual and consequently this kind of healing can be practiced only by persons who have the spiritual character. One must be spiritual in a prominent degree; he must also have lost sight of the thought of being an individual spirit. He must have lost sight of those feelings and brought himself into perfect harmony and unity with the Universal Spirit else he cannot do this kind of healing, and it is because of this fact that there are so few persons who really believe in Spiritual Healing. With the average person Spiritual Healing really means Psychical Healing — in many instances, Magnetic Healing, and very few realize that there is such a thing as healing which is performed by the Universal Spirit passing through the spirit of the healer into that of the patient.

Divine Healing differs from Spiritual Healing in that it is not the Universal Spirit, but the Divine Spirit, the Spiritus Sanctus, that is the Healing Force. In this case the same state of sympathy, harmony and unity must exist between the healer and the patient, but the healer himself must be functioning on the Maha-Para-Nirvanic Plane at the time he is accomplishing the healing. He must be in union with the Spirit of God so that it permeates his being and fills him. Thus he must identify himself with God. He must lose sight of all thought of self, all materiality and everything of that kind. His individuality must be entirely obliterated for the time being so that he is conscious of his absolute union with God. This can be accomplished only by Mystics of the highest order. When the Spirit of God flows through his being and acts upon the spirit of the patient and coming down, heals the various principles by bringing them into harmony with God, so that they are united and the connection is made between the Spirit of God and the Spirit of the patient and all the way down, when man has been brought into that state of perfect union with God, then the illness will naturally disappear and this is what it means to accomplish Divine Healing.

Let it be understood definitely that an atheist can never perform Divine Healing because he cannot bring himself into that state of sympathetic union with God. An infidel or a rationalist cannot do this kind of healing. He may be very spiritual in the sense of having considerable spirituality, but a person must have attained UNION with GOD before he can accomplish this kind of work. He may be a Para-Nirvani and yet if he sees nothing beyond the Universal Spirit he cannot do Divine Healing, because he cannot get in touch with this Spirit, he cannot get into harmony with it, and, therefore, cannot administer it to his patient.

It should be distinctly understood that the Divine Healer is one who is in a state of conscious union with the Spirit of God. By reason of this, the Spirit of God acts through his being, passes from him and thus enters into the organism of the patient, first acting upon his spirit and then down through the various principles of his being. For this reason no detrimental effects are ever found to result from Divine Healing. It is always beneficial and never otherwise. It is not the magnetism of the Healer that is used, but the Spirit of God; the vibration is all on the Divine Octave. However, of course, it has to be lowered to the lower octaves, as it comes down, otherwise the patient could not endure it, but it is purely divine in its origin and consequently cannot have any evil influence. Not only will it cure the body, but it also heals the spirit, the soul and the mind, the Astral body and everything of the kind. The Divine Healer is a physician of Souls as well as of bodies. Thus the vibration going on in the spirit will be in perfect harmony with the Spirit of God, and likewise, the soul, the Buddhic vibration, is brought into perfect harmony, the mind and the emotions, everything, are in harmony with God, so that at the expiration of a treatment the patient has a much clearer and a more spiritual mind, his reasoning is much deeper and more spiritual and his emotions are soon to be more spiritual, more and more in accordance with the Spirit of God and the eternal fitness of things and because of this fact, because he is brought into this state of being, this state of absolute harmony, we find that he is a better man by reason of having received the treatment, and it has been observed that those who have received the treatment, and that those who have received Spiritual Healing acquire a change of character to a great extent. It makes them better, brings them more into harmony with God and that is really the mission of the Divine Healer. He should not think of healing people simply to cure them of their bodily diseases. That is not his mission. He should make the healing of the body a means of healing the soul. However, in some instances this will be found to bring a very great degree of disturbance in the constitution of the patient because his emotions, for instance, are antagonistic to God, they are material or sensual or selfish; they are not in harmony with the Divine at all. Now, when a vibration which is in perfect harmony with the Divine Spirit, the Divine Vibration strikes the Astral Body, it begins to establish emotions of a spiritual character. These are antagonized by his normal emotional state. The result is a disturbance, a discordant state of emotion is brought about and it is likely to make the patient worse. He is liable to become sick as a result of his emotions, or he may get along distracted under the influence, and it is only by a tremendous current of the Divine Spirit coming with sufficient force to change the vibration completely, to neutralize all those influences and establish spiritual conditions in the emotional nature and its vehicle, that these disturbing influences can be overcome. Therefore, it is not advisable for healers to practice Divine Healing excepting in such cases as the patient really wants to become spiritual, where he really is anxious to get out of these improper emotional states, because if he antagonizes this spiritual influence

27

it will in many instances make him worse than otherwise, unless the person has a tremendous amount of spiritual force, so that he is able to entirely overcome this antagonistic state.

The Divine Healer, therefore, should heal only when requested to do so and should heal only when he is recognized as a Divine Healer. He should not allow himself to be classed as a Faith Doctor, or a magnetic healer, or anything of that kind. He should always hold himself forth as a Divine Healer, giving God the glory and forcing his patient to do likewise, that is recognize the Divine Force operating through him, the healer. In this way, if he maintain his religious character, his spiritual bases, and they come to him in this way, they are likely to recognize his position and thus bring their principles more into a susceptible state in reference to God and His Spirit. One whose mind is skeptical, rationalistic, materialistic in regard to God is by this very fact separated from and antagonistic to God's Spirit. His mind instead of being negative to the Spirit of God is positive, consequently it is very difficult to heal one who is antagonistic in this way. One who does not believe cannot easily be healed, not so much that faith is necessary, not so much that there is nothing but suggestion involved, but his attitude of unbelief will drive away, will repel the Spirit of God whereas belief has but little to do with magnetic healing.

But when Spiritual Healing does get in its work it really has the influence of changing his processes of thought, of changing his mental activity. One whose reason has been developed along lines away from the Spirit of God, is also antagonistic in a certain degree, but if this can be overcome so that the spirit is able to get in its work it has the effect not only of healing his body, but also of healing his soul, his spirit, his mind, his heart, and everything else, because it reaches the body only by reason of its already having accomplished the work in the higher principles. Thus the person will become a good man or a good woman, Godlike, saintly, as a result of these treatments, when they are given by a true Divine Healer.

Now, the Divine Healer must be in a state of Oneness with God in order to accomplish Divine Healing because he cannot otherwise get the Divine Power. It does not come to him unless there is a state of affinity existing between his own spirit and the Spirit of God. It is for this reason that healers must lead austere lives. They must lead lives wherein the spiritual principle becomes the predominating one, wherein the Spirit is the strongest force, at the same time it must be in perfect harmony with God's Spirit. They must keep His commandments and live in accordance with His word. They must be men of faith. They must have lost sight of the external and wordly thoughts and feelings and everything of that kind. No one but a saint can be a Divine Healer. Men and Women who are not saints, who claim to be divine healers are liars. They may perform magnetic healing, possibly psychical healing, but Divine Healing is an utter impossibility to one who is not a saint, and the highest perfection of Divine Healing is possible to a Christian only. A certain amount of it may be done by persons who have not become Christians, that is by a person who knows nothing about Christianity but is very devout, and spiritual, who recognizes the Divine Spirit and who has developed powers by contemplation and meditation, but it cannot in the highest sense be performed by any one but a Christian. Now, the man who does not know the difference between the Divine Spirit and the Universal Spirit is usually simply acting with the Universal Spirit. Of course, there are some persons who know nothing of nature, but only know the Divine Mysteries, who do not recognize any difference between the two, but the ordinary person who does not know the difference simply knows the Universal but not the Divine Spirit.

The Divine Healer fully recognizes his healing as being a religious act, as part of his spiritual ministration and as being a gift from God. However, one who is not by nature a good psychical healer can never be a good Divine Healer, or a Divine Healer of any kind, for that matter and the reason of this is quite plain, quite simple if you look at it properly. The Divine Spirit supplies the Healing Force in Divine Healing, gives the same as in Psychical Healing, consequently a person must be able to do psychical healing, plus the Spirit of God in order to do Divine Healing. Spiritual Healing is Psychical Healing plus the Universal Spirit. Now, when one has received the Holy Spirit if he was already a healer, then the capacity to heal, or the Spirit of God will naturally flow through that channel, will naturally express itself in that way, but if he does not have the capacity, then it will express itself in some other way, so do not for a moment get the idea that a person's being in harmony with the Spirit of God, in union with the Divine Spirit must necessarily confer upon him healing power. He must be a healer already if it does. He will have a spiritual power, but it depends upon the character of his make-up, the faculties and powers that he had already as to the channel through which this Spirit will flow, will operate, and in order to accomplish a great deal of this work, it is necessary that he confine himself almost exclusively to it; also he should not try to practice any other kind of healing when he begins to do Divine Healing. He should abandon all other methods and let the Spirit of God act upon his patient. Another thing, he should never heal a person who is not willing to have his soul and spirit healed as well as his body.

The Divine Healer when he takes a patient should look to see if the disease has come upon the patient as a result of any sin which he has committed, any special sin, and if so, he should heal him only on condition that he repent of the sin. A person should be healed only on condition that he should renounce all his sins and if he does not do it, if he gets diseased a second time he should not be healed at all, but allowed to rot or die or anything else. He should be healed only once for the same disease, and this should be on condition that he will repent of his sins. As Jesus said "Thy sins be forgiven thee," whenever He healed disease, so the Divine Healer should regard himself as a Priest whose mission it is to forgive sins, therefore, he should never heal until he has first shown the patient that his disease has come as a punishment for sins, that it is caused by certain sins that he has committed. He should bring this home to the patient and should not give him a single treatment unless the patient admits it - that is in a case where the sickness has come as a result of sin and not because of accident or anything of that kind. We are speaking now of those diseases which are the result of sin either against God's revealed Law or His Natural Law. Now when one realizes this and admits it, confesses that he has sinned, he should then be required to abandon those sins and having repented of his sins the Divine Healer should heal him of his diseases, free him from the consequences of those sins which he has now abandoned.

This is really the work of the Divine Healer and he should work to that end, always recognizing the fact that he is not a physician of bodies alone, but a physician of souls that he is a priest as well as a doctor and he should never allow himself to be classed as a physician, but always as a priest. In the Divine Healer we have the priestly physician applied in a therapeutic way. The person who will not recognize him in his priestly capacity, who does not have faith, should not be given the benefit of his offices, should not be healed unless some one else comes and intercedes and supplies the faith, — a member of his family or some one closely related to him.

It should also be borne in mind that it is possible for a Divine Healer to heal people without placing his hands on their faculties this being merely a convenience and an important aid, but the healing can be affected without touching the patient, simply by projecting this spiritual power, this Divine Force from the organism of the Healer into that of his patient, or by calling it down and transmitting it, so that the Aura of the patient is entirely permeated by this healing force. Likewise he may heal at long distances without having touched the patient in the slightest degree, even being hundreds or thousands of miles from him, there being no limit to the distance over which the Spirit of God travels.

But we may briefly sum up the nature of Divine Healing by saying it is the Spirit of God applied through the organism of a Healer who is in harmony with God and in sympathy with the patient, to the patient's principles and ultimately to his body, for the purpose of bringing about a state of health and harmony, and it is applied in the same way that all other healing forces are applied. In Magnetic Healing it is the animal magnetism that is applied; in Psychical Healing, the psychical force of the healer, and in Spiritual Healing the Universal Spirit, so in Divine Healing it is the Spirit of God, and the means employed in bringing this Spirit of God into contact with the patient, enabling it to transform the being of the patient, are the same means as those employed in any other kind of healing. Being, however, of a higher rate of vibration, on a higher octave, it is, therefore, much more powerful in its action than any of the other healing agents, — likewise being of a much finer vibration, it is possible to charge the body of the patient with a far greater quantity of this force than with any of the lower principles. What would cause pain, severe shock, even disruption to the body if magnetism were employed, will cause no disturbance at all when the Spirit of God is applied. It being of so much finer vibration, will admit a much more powerful current without any danger whatsoever to the patient. However, it may not be at all best for one whose passions are violent and one whose ambitions are of a vile or gross character to receive a current of the Spirit of God. There are persons of such character that there would be danger of their being struck dead the moment they received a current of the Spirit of God, because of their bitter antagonism, their opposition to those emotional vibrations, etc., which will be awakened and set up whenever the Spirit of God comes in contact with their spirits, and their lower principles. For such, it is best to shun the Divine Healer, — it is best for them to resort to healing agents of a lower potency, but for the one who is able to come into harmony with God's Spirit, is able to become negative to it and yield to its transforming influence, so that the chemical processes necessary may go on within his being, there is nothing so advantageous as Divine Healing.

LESSON
ON
ABSENT HEALING

As the healing force is not limited by space, but being a cosmic principle, may go to any distance, in the same way electricity or magnetism or anything else would go, it follows logically that healing may be accomplished at a considerable distance from the healer. We do not have to be in personal contact with the patient in order to accomplish the work of healing. Absent Treatment is quite as practical in its operation, as treatment by contact; in fact we find the principle of Absent Treatment is employed by a number of healers who do not call themselves Absent Healers. For instance quite often the healer cures his patients without touching them; that is to say, he gives his treatments without placing his hands upon the patients. The method of the Christian Scientist is solely an application of the Absent Practice. The Healer sits by the patient and concentrates in his own mind and while, of course, they call it the realization of the illusion of diseases and everything of that kind, the reality of Spirit, nevertheless the healer is transmitting healing force to the organism of his patient by reason of the realization of the picture, — it is by Mental picturing that the work is really accomplished. The healing force is transmitted to the patient by reason of the transmission of the vibratory state; that is to say, the rate of vibration operative within the Aura of the Healer is transmitted to the Aura of the patient and this accomplishes the work.

Healers quite often accomplish works of healing without touching their patient, without the patient knowing that he is being healed. The only thing to do is to simply form the mental picture and go through the manner of healing in the same way you would by contact, only you do not put your hands upon the patient, because magnetism, psychical force, or spiritual force, as the case may be, may be transmitted through the Aura or Ether from one organism to another, therefore, healing may be accomplished without coming into physical contact with the patient.

32

Now, if you can heal a person across a room, without touching him while standing at the opposite side of the room, on the same principle you can heal him at a distance of a thousand miles. There are several methods which may be followed, any one of which will be found to be very effective. In the first place, you may sit quietly, enter the silence, and form in mind a picture of your patient sitting before you just as though he were there in the room, and then you begin to transmit the current. Follow the rule exactly the same in this treatment that you do in the ordinary treatment. If you are going to practice magnetic healing, you should fix your attention upon your patient and will for your magnetism to go to him and enter his body and as it passes down the spinal cord, it will go out along the proper nerves until it reaches the part, and there magnetize it just the same way you would if you were giving a magnetic treatment, the only difference being that you do not touch the person with your hands. Of course, you could not do that as he is at a considerable distance from you. Simply will for your magnetism to enter his body and then, by concentration of the will, direct the attention along the nerves the way the current is to go, keeping in mind the picture of the magnetism flowing along and doing this work; at the same time keeping in mind the picture of the transformation which is to take place. Now, if you will do this with sufficient concentration, you will be able to accomplish the relief of any disease, by magnetism.

On the other hand, you may want to treat a functional disease, or some organic trouble, something which requires the magnetizing of the sympathetic nerves. In that case you want to fix your attention on the Solar Plexus, of your patient; then will for a current of magnetism to flow into the Solar Plexus, filling it up and charging it with a magnetic force. Then let it flow out along the sympathetic nerves, so that they are quickened, stimulated and magnetized, until you come to the nerve center that is weak. If it be a functional disease, all you have to do is to magnetize this nerve center sufficiently to enable it to perform its proper functions. When it has thus been sufficiently magnetized, the treatment is over for the time being. Give your treatments regularly just the same as you would if the patient were coming to you. Stimulate his nerve center until it has finally gained the necessary strength to perform the functions in a proper manner. While stimulating a nerve center you should always hold in mind a picture of the result you wish to accomplish. That is, if you want to treat the heart in this way, see the heart beating in just the proper manner. See it performing its functions properly. If you are treating any stomach trouble, see the stomach digesting the food, see it in a state of perfect health, direct it in its activities, and at the same time keep this magnetic current flowing in there by watching it flow in. Your magnetic force is sent through the Aura to the place

33

where your patient is in, the same way that the vibration of Hertzian waves are sent forth through the ether, in wireless telegraphy. You direct this force so that it flows to your patient.

Now, observe this point carefully, it is not by _thinking_ that we heal. There is no gerater error than to assume that man accomplishes healing by thinking. You may think all you want to for your patient but you are not going to transmit healing magnetism by thought. It is by a concentration of the will that the healing force is sent. You may not know how to heal, but if your will is exercised in precisely the right direction, you will find you will be able to heal your patient in a remarkable manner. The will is the positive pole of the emotions; it represents Desire positively expressed. By this statement it will be understood what is to be done in healing. It is not simply to think, not simply to talk to the patient in a way, but it is to COMMAND, that is the force which heals; it is the Word of Command.

You may practice Psychical Healing in the same way you do Magnetic Healing; that is to say, you may concentrate the attention upon the faculty of Spirituality of your patient and thus follow the same method that you do in the regular Psychical Healing when you have your hands on the patient. You do all the work of control by concentration of the attention. It is not absolutely necessary to concentrate on this Organ of Spirituality at all. You may make a picture of the patient in all his entirety, that is, you may picture him with his Aura permeating his body and see within the seven principles of his being. Now, when you have concentrated upon these seven principles, fix your attention specifically upon his Soul; transmit the healing current to his soul principle and then let it go down to the lower principles, on down until it acts upon the psychical body in the same way you would practice ordinarily when giving Psychical Healing.

If you want to practice Spiritual Healing, you follow the same rule, only concentrating upon his Spirit and transmit, by the focusing of the attention, your own spiritual force, so that the patient is made to receive it; his spirit is charged with it. Then you go on down, descending from one principle to another until at last you act upon the particular part which is diseased, forming in mind a picture of what you want to take place, seeing it actually taking place, actually transpiring. When you have done that you will accomplish the work.

In all these methods of healing, the Law of Periodicity should be observed; that is to say you should have certain days on which you give the treatments and never fail to give the treatment on that day, providing you are not giving the treatments every day.

You should also have a specific hour, even to the moment, to give the treatment. If the patient knows you are treating him, it is best to have him also observe the same time and at the moment when the treatment is to begin, sit or lie quietly in his room, relaxing every muscle, relaxing the mind and spirit and wait in a receptive attitude, an attitude of expectancy, waiting for the operation of the healing force, and also it is a good idea to have him concentrate his mind in this passive way, upon the seat of the disease, and hold in mind the picture of the healing work; see the healing force operative there; in other words, he should co-operate with you in the treatment, only he should be negative while you are positive. When you have a patient, who is capable of this negative co-operation with you, you will have but little difficulty in curing him.

You may practice Suggestive Therapeutics at a distance, as well as these other forms of healing, and to do this, all that is necessary is to form in your imagination a picture of your patient and then, by concentrating the mind, simply talk to him, simply give the suggestion in the same way; also give it as though you had him right before you. Even suppose you want to give a person suggestive treatment in the room where you are. You can do it much better by thinking than by speaking. Simply form in your mind the thoughts which you wish to transmit, keeping your mind positive and you will project them to his mind. Now in the same way, you may concentrate and positively transmit your thought to one who is thousands of miles removed from you, giving him a suggestion, telling him just what to do, telling him just what is going to take place and he will respond in the same way he would respond if you were talking to him.

You may also practice Divine Healing at a distance. This is accomplished by drawing into your own being the power of God, the Divine Spirit, and at the same time remaining in perfect harmony with your patient, realizing your unity with him, merging your very identity into that of your patient, and while maintaining this state of deep concentration realize the inflowing of the Spirit of God into his body, see it flowing in there. Form the spiritual realization and while maintaining this state of spiritual realization, this spiritual concentration, you will be transmitting the force to the body of your patient. Observe however, that to do this properly you must be positive to the patient in the same way you would in the other methods of treatment. The key to the situation in the maintenance of a state of negative concentration with reference to God and positive concentration with reference to your patient, so that by being negative you attain to Oneness with God and thus through that, with the Spirit, and by maintaining a positive state of harmony with your patient, you transmit the healing potency to his organism.

It is necessary that you observe the state of absolute union at all times when giving treatments by any of these methods.

If your patient knows you are treating him, have him concentrate at the same time, and he should concentrate by observing an attitude of expectancy, coupled with one of powerful desire. You, on the other hand, should concentrate the Will powerfully in the most positive manner, thus projecting the force to your patient. However, it is possible to accomplish healing without the patient knowing anything about it. In this way you can do a great deal of work that you could not do by any other method. It is always, however, much easier to transmit the healing force to one who is co-operating with you than to one who does not know anything about the work. Do not get the idea, however, that you can accomplish as much, that is to say, as great results by the same treatment at long distance as you could if your patient were with you and you were giving him direct applications of the healing power. You cannot do this, for the simple reason that the power diminishes according to the distance it has to travel. A certain amount of the healing force is scattered. It requires the concentration of the Will to project magnetism to any distance at all, and its general tendency is to diffuse itself through space. To make it travel a direct line to concentrate a powerful current to a given point, it becomes absolutely necessary that we should concentrate the Will with considerable force. In this way we will keep the magnetism or the Spirit whatever it is, together, thus concentrating a powerful stream of this force instead of diffusing it over a great deal of space. In fact, the difference between the Healer and the other man is not so much in the fact that the Healer has a large quantity of magnetism, as it is his ability to concentrate his force on a given point and force this to flow in a concentrated stream while the other man scatters his forces and thus does not accomplish any very great results upon any one point. The principle, therefore, in the healing power consists of the one-pointedness of concentration. This is particularly true of Absent Treatment, but as this one-pointedness so far as the transmitted force is concerned, is gradually lost as it travels, because the power of concentration diminishes in strength according to the square of the distance, the result will be that man who could perform wonders at a short distance, will have no effect at a distance of a hundred or a thousand miles. It is best, therefore, that we should not practice Absent Treatment if we can have the patient come to us, it being much better to have him with us, than to undertake to treat him at a distance but where this cannot be done, where we cannot have the patient with us, it is advisable to practice Absent Treatment.

It requires much greater concentration upon the part of the healer to accomplish results in the absent way than to accomplish them by the direct treatment, consequently there is more work for him and he is entitled to just as much, in fact, to a greater compensation than in cases in which he gives them direct, although he cannot accomplish the same results.

Absent Treatment, is therefore, the application of the same fundamental principles that are employed in the direct treatment. The

Healer should bear in mind that the method is precisely the same, the only difference being that it is by fixing the attention and by positive concentration of the Will that the work is accomplished by Absent Treatment. This is also the way in which we heal by direct treatment, only in direct treatment we use the hands, come in direct contact with the patient's body, while in absent treatment we transmit the healing force through the atmosphere or the ether, and thus come in contact with the organism of the patient, the ether acting as the plastic medium through which the healing force passes from one organism to another.

The analogy between Absent Treatment and Wireless Telegraphy is almost perfect. If you assume that the Hertzian waves transmitted in wireless telegraphy represent the Healing Magnetism employed in Absent Treatment, then the analogy will be perfect, the ether in either case being the plastic medium between the two instruments, the vibration being the same, that is, as it passes through this plastic medium exercising a corresponding influence upon the organism of the patient.

Absent Treatment is, therefore, not a figment of the imagination, not an illusion, not a mystical vagary, but is an application of the known laws of physics to the healing of the body at a distance from the healer, its laws being the same as any other methods of Healing, but of course, its potency not so great as that of the ordinary healing methods, because it naturally diminishes in accordance with the square of the distance that the force has to travel.

LESSON
ON
HIGH POTENCY HOMEOPATHY

One of the departments of material medicine, High Potency Homeopathy, is, in reality, metaphysical in its fundamental principles. The vibratory law, which governs in all departments of metaphysical therapeutics, is really the fundamental principle operative in the high potency system.

The fundamental principle of Homeopathy is the active principle, the spirit, so to speak, of the drug, which must be extracted and employed. The crude drug, the body of the drug, is to be avoided, and the only way known to the Homeopath, to get rid of the body of the drug is by attenuation, so the method is to attenuate the drug to the lowest possible point. In so doing, the percentage of the crude drug will be rendered correspondingly low, while the spirit of the drug remains, and this will exercise its influence upon the system unto the purging out the diseased condition.

However, it is not orthodox Homeopathy we are interested in just now, but the high potency branch of the school. The principle of High Potency Homeopathy is the trituration of the drug and if we look at it properly we will see that they are really making use of the vibratory law. In making trituration, nine parts of sugar to one part of the drug are placed together. Then while the trituration is being made it is stirred with a glass rod a certain number of times; say a hundred times. Then they place one part of that to nine parts of sugar and make a second trituration, stirring a hundred times. The first trituration is 1x. The second is 2x. Each further trituration is one-tenth of the first added to nine parts of sugar. Some of the high potency homeopaths make as high as 30x. That means the thirtieth attenuation, or in plain English one-third of one per cent of the drug and ninety-nine and two-thirds per cent sugar. In those thirty attenuations it has been stirred a hundred times each or three thousand times in making the trituration.

Now, as a matter of fact, it is the stirring that really accomplishes the work. You can readily see that after a drug has gone through thirty attenuations there would not be any curative efficacy in it, from the standpoint of ordinary pharmacy. It is not its chemical character, but the stirring that makes the remedy, and bear in mind, the most powerful drugs, so far as their therapeutic value is concerned, are these very triturations, these very potentized remedies. As the rod is triturating the remedy it is held in the hand of the triturator and his attention is fixed, is concentrated upon the object in hand. He is forming a picture all the time of the result he wishes to attain. He has before him the picture of certain effects which he wishes to produce. He is undertaking to cure his patient of a certain disease; he must bring about certain physiological results and, for this reason, he has in mind the image of the picture that is to be produced on the same principle as any other mental picturing. He does not have to know anything about the law of mental picturing, though most of the high potency Homeopaths do have an inkling of it, but the very fact of his keeping his mind concentrated on the result which he wishes to accomplish, keeps that picture clearly in his consciousness, and as he continues to hold this picture, the Aura is made to vibrate in harmony with it. The picture establishes the corresponding vibration throughout his Aura. All those whirls which correspond to the picture are there established. His Mental Body is vibrating continually and expressing that picture, and as it descends to the Astral Body it also receives the vibration and responds to it, so that that picture is expressing itself continually in the Astral. The Astral, in turn, acts upon the Etheric Double and causes it to vibrate in tune with the vibration of the Astral. The picture is thus expressed in the vibration of the Etheric Double. This last, in turn, acts upon the gross physical body, causing the nerve currents to flow in harmony, and the entire circulation of the nervous system is thus expressing the picture which is held in the consciousness, acting in harmony with it. The nerves, in turn, stimulate the muscles to contract and relax according to the shifting character of the picture. The result is, the motions of the body or muscles, are the very expression of this mental picture, and because of this muscular contraction and relaxation, which is the very same principle which is found operative in muscle reading, the trained muscle reader simply sensing the muscular contraction and relaxation. This causes the fingers to tremble and quiver according to the impulse that is flowing from the picture. Every tremor, every quiver of the hand is but the expression, but the outward manifestation of that vibrating force, which is, in turn, the expression of the picture. By holding a pen in the fingers, the tremor, the quiver of the fingers is imparted to it, thus determining the formation of the letters. It is in this way that by graphology, it

39

is possible to diagnose a person's thoughts at the time he is writing, his feelings, to know the picture which is in his consciousness, by the formation of the letters. Likewise if we get the mean of those eccentricities in the formation of the letters, we will be able to estimate his character because we can see what is continuously in his consciousness, what is governing his vibration, etc. Now, it is in the same way that by holding a glass rod in the hand, the vibration expressing itself through the quiver of the hand, is imparted to the rod and it, in turn, quivers, trembles, and vibrates as the hand moves. Therefore, the body of the rod is the perfect ego, so to speak, of the man, of the combination which is the expression of the muscular man, and all being the effect of the picture held in the consciousness.

Now, as this picture represents the effect which is to be produced, it consequently generates or establishes the rate of vibration which will be present in that effect. The picture of health, for instance, will establish a healthy vibration and thus it is passed down through the various media, the Astral body, the Etheric Double, etc., the nerves, muscles, and everything, all along until that glass rod, responding to that vibration, generating the same vibration, will impart to the solution, the same rate of vibration and cause it to vibrate accordingly.

Now, every time an attenuation is made it has been stirred a hundred times and all the time during the stirring, the rod is vibrating. It has the same effect in a general way that the electric vibrator would have on a person or anything of the kind. It is continually vibrating and as the stirring goes on more and more of this vibration is imparted to the solution, and as the attenuations are made from time to time, there is less and less of the drug and more and more of the vibration. The result is, when the last attenuation is made, the result is not a drug at all but is in reality, a bottled up vibration and is powerfully charged in this way and quite as effectively charged as by sending a current of electricity through it.

It should be borne in mind that the therapeutic value of the trituration depends upon the intensity of the concentration. The more perfectly the picture is held in mind, and consequently the more intensely the vibration is concentrated there, the more powerfully will it become the embodiment of that vibration, consequently the more efficacious it will become as a therapeutic agent. Also, we must bear in mind the imagination and its wonderful influence. A person who is not imaginative should never triturate a medicine. One who looks at everything from a common sense standpoint will accomplish but few results. The man with a vivid imagination, the one able to make very vivid, clear pictures and to hold them for a considerable length of time, the one who is enthusiastic about the work, who feels he is going to accomplish results, who wants to help people, can accomplish much more than another can, because the picture is far more vivid and, therefore, his vibration is far more intense. He is breathing health into the solution all the time he is making the trituration.

The higher the potency or trituration, the less of the drug there is in it. It is the quantity of sugar and, consequently the number of times it has been stirred, the amount of trituration, that establishes the potency of the trituration. The High Potency physician, therefore, considers medicine stronger, more powerful in proportion as it has been triturated, and that means attenuated, — not in proportion to the presence of the drug. It is, therefore, the vibration that counts, but this vibration will be in proportion to the vividness of the imagination and to the degree of concentration.

We should not fall into the error of thinking that the potency depends merely upon the number of attenuations, upon the length of time the trituration has lasted. It depends much more upon the man who is doing the triturating. Likewise, it depends largely upon the general character of the man's vibration. That must be taken into consideration. One who is habitually healthy, whose entire attitude is one of health, will naturally have a healthy vibration, and that will be imparted to the trituration. Further, one who believes in health, one who is optimistic will have a general vibration of this kind and that will be involved. Further, if the man have a specific disease the vibration of that disease will be imparted to the remedy while the trituration is going on, so that instead of its being a curative agent it will effectually inoculate the patient with a certain disease. No person should ever attempt to triturate a remedy unless he is perfectly free from disease, unless he is optimistic and in a healthy frame of mind, unless his whole attitude is in accord with health.

Another thing: there are certain characteristics of mind, certain faculties and certain propensities which have a corresponding rate of vibration, and one having an undesirable propensity should never triturate, because he will impart that vibration, so that the influence of that upon his body will be communicated directly to the body of his patient, through the remedy. A person should never triturate when he is out of sorts, or angry, when his mind is not in a state of perfect harmony. He should always be in a state of absolute calm, of poise, so that he will impart that poise, that calm vibration. If he is not in such state, he should not attempt to make a trituration.

It will, therefore, be readily seen how important it is that only the right kind of a person should perform a trituration, in order that a perfectly normal, proper vibration alone may be imparted, the potentized remedy thus becoming the physical vehicle for the impartation of vibration.

41

The high potency Homeopaths have recognized the vibratory character of their remedies to the extent that they have required that in all potentized remedies the entire trituration shall be made by one person; no one shall take his place after it has begun; the same one must complete the trituration, and this is evidently for the purpose of preventing different magnetisms acting upon it, different vibrations; so that it may have the same vibration all the way through; but this will not prevent a weak vibration being imparted by one whose vibration is naturally weak.

We can readily see from the admission that is here made by the regulations, so far as they were able to make them, that the value of an attenuation or trituration depends absolutely upon the man who is making it. No man who is not qualified to heal magnetically and psychically is qualified to make a trituration. We should, therefore, realize that the fundamental principles of Vibratory Therapeutics are also the fundamental principles of High Potency Homeopathy. We are really employing identical systems, and all the way through; it is the application of the great vibratory law, the only difference being that we realize the high potency homeopaths impart vibration to a physical medium and use that as a means of communicating a vibration to the body of the patient and the Metaphysical Healers use some metaphysical medium for the same purpose, such as magnetism or psychical force or something of that kind, the Suggestive Therapeutists employ suggestion for the same purpose, to impart the vibration to the minds of the patients. In other words, the secret of the healing art is the impartation of the healing vibration to the patient's Aura; that is what really accomplishes the cure. You may impart that directly to the Aura, as in Magnetic Healing and Psychical Healing and such methods, or you may impart it through the formation of a mental picture in the patient's consciousness, by Suggestion, or in the third place, you may form the mental picture in your own mind so as to establish the vibration within your own Aura and then transmit that vibration to a physical medium, as in the high potency method, forming a potentized remedy which is the material channel through which the vibration is imparted to the patient's Aura. In either case, however, it is vibration that is employed for establishing the state of health, health being an harmonious state of vibration, and disease a discordant state of vibration. Healing consists in replacing the discordant vibration with harmonious vibration, Harmony of Vibration, therefore, being a therapeutic agent. Mental Picturing is the force which regulates the character of the vibration. High Potency Homeopathy is, therefore, an application of this law to therapeutic uses, by establishing the vibration in a physical agent and using that as the connection between the healer and the Aura of his patient.

LESSON
ON
CHRISTIAN SCIENCE

The Christian Science System of metaphysical therapeutics begins with the assumption of two minds, what they term the mortal mind and the immortal mind. Disease is supposed to be due to the errors of mortal mind; the thinking of the mortal mind, being erroneous, sows the seeds of discord which result in disease. Immortal mind, on the contrary, is always healthful; its thinking is promotive of harmony and therefore, will establish health.

The entire system of Christian Science as a healing system is in reality the replacing of suggestions or thoughts of mortal mind with those of the immortal mind. A treatment consists in a course of instruction from the point of view of the immortal mind and a denial of the errors of mortal mind.

It is difficult to ascertain just what they mean by these expressions, but when we get at the foundation, we see that their system is perfectly true and of the very highest order. Very few Scientists have ever realized what is meant by those expressions, — as a matter of fact they mean by Mortal Mind, the Human Mind; every thought of the human mind is mortal and is, therefore, promotive of disease. By the immortal mind they mean the Divine Mind, the God Mind. Now, mortal mind thinks erroneously; its thought is always untrue; it is out of harmony with the Divine Mind and because of this discordant state, it expresses itself in discordant vibration, disturbing forces, which shut us off from the higher life force. We are told by Scientists that sickness, sin, pain and death are all errors of the mortal mind, and in the highest metaphysical sense, this is literally true, but unfortunately, we do not realize the metaphysical usuage often enough. Too many people are prone to assume this to be a literal statement of facts from the standpoint of the physical. The action of the mortal or human mind is really error because it is in opposition to the Divine Mind. The Divine Mind is always true; its thinking, its emotions are the expression of the highest truth and as it moves, as it thinks, the vibration is set up which will express health, life, happiness, etc.

Christian Science recognizes that all activities of the human mind, or mortal mind, being antagonistic to the activities of the Divine Mind, must therefore, be erroneous in the sense of being out of harmony or antagonistic to that which is fundamental because the human mind deals with effects and not with causes and takes those effects for causes, assuming that they are fundamental, assuming that those appearances are realities. It, therefore, deals in the realm of Maya, from the Oriental point of view. Dealing in that realm, it is erroneous, it is illusory. Now, this is the true sense in which mortal mind is sowing errors, in which all the activities of the human mind are called the errors of mortal mind. It is in the dealing with the phenomenal and taking that for the real. The activities of the Divine Mind must generate in the being those vibratory effects, those emotions which are the effect of the Divine. In other words, those emotions of harmony must take the place of emotions, of discord, consequently if you can stop the thinking in this Maya, if you can stop this limited, phenomenal, illusory, thinking, and think from the standpoint of absolute reality, think always in universals, not in particulars, if you can think in abstract principles, think from the standpoint of the Divine Oneness, you will thus set aside all those emotions which are generated through the individualism of human thinking. Mortal mind then will cease to act and Immortal Mind will be acting because the Manas will now move under the impulse of Immortal Mind, duplicating those emotions, reproducing those thoughts, because it will simply be the embodying of the Divine Mind, letting that shine through the human. Manas, instead of being self-acting, will now be acted upon by the mind of God. It is this, that the Christian Scientists mean by replacing the errors of mortal mind by the truths of immortal mind — what they call immortal mind is the mind of God, acting upon and through the human mind, instead of the human mind directing its thinking. The human mind becoming the channel for the expression of the Divine Mind, is Immortal Mind; when it is self-acting, it is mortal; when this Immortal Mind has been established in opposition to or in the place of the mortal mind it will, therefore, establish the vibration of harmony throughout the system. Discord will be replaced by harmony and thus health will be the result. Sickness being the effect of discord which is the result of mortal mind thinking, will now be replaced by health, the effect of harmonious vibration, which is the result of Immortal Mind thinking.

Thus the natural consequences of the establishment of Immortal Mind in the place of Mortal Mind in the person's thinking, must necessarily be the establishment of perfect health in place of sickness.

Sickness is, therefore, shown to be the result of incorrect thinking, or thinking from the limited or human point of view; health must necessarily flow as naturally from correct thinking, thinking of a harmonious character, thinking which is the outgrowth of the immortal mind.

The perfect cure for all disease, then, is the establishment of the Divine Mind in and through the human. There is no other way to perfectly accomplish a permanent state of health, and in this they are right, for if we cure disease either by medicine, healing or any other way, and do not change the trend of one's thought, we allow the patient to continue in that individualistic road, to continue under the dominance of mortal mind and he will continue to sow the seeds of disease and his system will get sick again; but if his thinking can be regenerated, if he can be brought to think from the point of view of Immortal Mind, that is, if God's mind can operate through him, he will then think in a Cosmos instead of in a chaos and the result will be his body will be well, harmony will reign and perfect health; and the success which the Christian Scientists have accomplished has been due to the fact that they have succeeded in establishing harmony of vibration throughout the system of their patients. They also teach that sin is a consequence of the errors of mortal mind, and it is a fact that if man did not follow his own mind, if he allowed God's mind to operate through his, of course, he would not commit any sin. Death is also an error of mortal mind, that is death comes upon man because of his following his own mind, the human mind instead of the Divine Mind, but when the Divine Mind has become generally individualized by man, death will depart. That is all perfectly true.

But it is the therapeutic side of Christian Science that we are interested in at present. Those therapeutic effects are brought about by the establishing of universal harmony within the body. The method of treatment is the recognition that disease is an error of mortal mind. It is to emphasize that in the absolute, the eternal, there is no such thing as disease, and this is really an upsetting of an old error into which humanity has fallen, namely that sickness, sin and death and everything of that kind are fundamental; that they are absolutely necessary and that we should not look for anything else. The idea that it is possible to get beyond that, has been lost sight of, and so the Scientist practitioner would impress upon the mind of the patient the idea that all his sufferings are due to the fact that he is not living in the absolute; that he is living in the relative, and should see that in the absolute there is no such thing; that in the fundamental principles of nature disease does not exist; that disease is a discordant condition and is caused by being out of harmony with the fundamental and that if he will get in touch with the fundamental he will escape disease and everything of that kind. For this reason,

45

the Scientist tells the patient that there is no such thing as the disease he thinks he has; that is to say, it does not exist in the eternal; it is not real; it is the outgrowth of man's thinking; it is not a part of the world of God; disease is not a creation of God, but a creation of man, and for this reason it is transitory; it will pass away; and the Scientist tries to induce the patient to place his consciousness in that which is eternal, that which God has produced, and living in that, he places himself on a plane above and beyond all these things. Disease now cannot reach him because he is living in the realm of the real, not in the realm of the illusory which is the product of human thinking. That if you will cease your human thinking, you will place yourself on a plane where human thought cannot reach you, or where the effects of human thought cannot reach you, and that this is also the way to escape from disastrous suggestions; all those suggestions which are undesirable which flow from man's malicious mental malpractice immediately lose all their force when we have the Divine Mind operative within us. When we do this, the human mind having ceased to act, all those things coming from human mind cannot influence us.

The message of CHRISTIAN SCIENCE, therefore, is to establish the operation of the Divine Mind within us and in this way escape the influence of the human mind, the influence of all human thinking, and disease, being an effect of human thinking will no longer reach us; it will cease to exist for us, because disease is a consequence of human thought; that when human thought has ceased, disease ceases to be; to us it does not exist, and so the Healer teaches the patient that it is non-existent; teaches its illusory character and the method is usually, to teach that it has no existence at all, that it is all an illusion, to get the patients to realize, to form this higher ideal, so that the mental picture is formed of the ideal condition; to place that before the patient as a reality, and let him think in the terms of the Divine. Let his human mind reach out and flow towards the Divine point of view and in time, the DIVINE MIND WILL BE ENTHRONED. That is the idea, and if you take the suggestions that are offered to the patient of the Scientist, they are really suggestions designed for the purpose of establishing these divine principles. For instance, they say there is no sin, there is no disease, that God is good and God is all; all is good. These abstractions are stated, and all the thinking of the patient is supposed to be built up out of these abstractions. When one learns to think in the abstract instead of in the concrete, he will, therefore, get into harmony with the Universal Consciousness. Of course, in their effort to go beyond the relative, to think in the terms of the universal they run to the opposite extreme of failing to admit the relative existence of the relative, quite often, and so they go too far to the extreme, nevertheless they have the fundamental idea correct.

This line of suggestion which the Christian Scientist is continually offering, has the tendency to establish a mental picture of ideal conditions, and the picture will have the effect of establishing the proper rates of vibration within the system; will in other words, establish harmony.

The entire treatment is for the purpose of establishing pictures of harmony in the mind of the patient and thus give harmonious vibration throughout his Aura, establishing the state of harmony and leading up to harmonize thinking so as to bring the patient out of his state of discord. The Christian Scientist makes use of affirmations and denials as means of establishing this picture. In order to build up the picture and to keep it in mind, the patient is instructed to affirm, I am so and so; that is, affirm those things which are regarded as being the teachings of Immortal Mind; to continually affirm the thoughts of Immortal Mind, to identify himself with the Immortal Mind, to affirm all the suggestions coming from that mind and thus he will picture the Immortal Mind within himself; will reflect that within his mind; that by denying the suggestions of Mortal Mind they can be kept out, that we can drive them out by denying them; — and here they make a FATAL MISTAKE. All the weaknesses and failures in Christian Science are due, principally to this practice of denials. It should not be indulged in, under any consideration. By denying anything we form a picture of it just as effectively as we do by affirming it. It is not our belief in a thing, that injures us, but the picture of the thing which we have in mind, because that picture attracts the vibration; it is the force back of the vibration, which is expressing itself through vibration. This force which vibrates throughout the system, being the cause of the physical condition, the cause of health and disease and being regulated and determined by the pictures in mind, depends upon the degree of those pictures for its therapeutic effect. Our opinion of those pictures has absolutely no effect. A picture of disease must set up the vibration which will express itself in disease, while a picture of health must express the vibration of health, our intellectual view of those pictures having no influence upon their effects. The only value of correct opinions is the influence they have in the establishment of correct pictures in the mind. Our thinking is, therefore, the cause of the pictures that we have before us continually and they establish the state of health. The affirmations of health and positive condition are likewise valuable because they are setting up those positive vibrations which will express themselves in healthy states, but to deny a disease, a specific disease, particularly, is to form a picture of that condition in the subconscious, and to form such a picture means to set up the vibration corresponding to it; that is the vibration which will actually exist in that disease, and thus to embody it.

Christian Science with the denials left out, simply resorting to the affirmations is a perfectly logical system of therapeutics. In fact it is one of the highest forms, depending as it does, upon the establishment of the Divine Mind in the place of the human, as a means of establishing harmony and therefore, health.

Another error which they have made is in discarding natural methods of healing, in repudiating hygiene and everything of the kind and teaching they may by simply living in the consciousness of the Divine, by having the Divine Mind manifest through him, would be able to maintain perfect health and need not pay any attention to his physical living. This, of course, is an error. We should live as near perfection as possible; we should conform our lives all the way through to the highest point of purity and by so doing we will remove a great deal of work which must be done by the changing of the thought. Then let us think in harmony with the Divine, let Immortal Mind take the place of Mortal Mind, but at the same time do not discount the importance of correct physical living. Of course, the error alluded to, grows out of the idealism which Mrs. Eddy taught, namely that man is spirit and being a spirit, is not dependent upon matter, that there are no material influences which can be brought to bear upon the human spirit, consequently, we should not pay any attention to these things, that if we go to resorting to hygiene and material agents we are thus placing ourselves on a material basis, we are thus recognizing the material, and thus descending to the plane of mortal mind; that we should bear in mind that we are not material, but are spirit and being spirit, matter cannot have any influence upon us. But this is an error, due to a failure to realize the fact that material things are just as spiritual as we are. Did they realize that everything, that matter itself, is simply spirit on a lower octave, then all these difficulties would be removed. They fail to realize this, thinking that all is an illusion, failing to recognize the reality of the physical body, and of course, in one sense its unreality is true, the body is not real in the highest metaphysical sense, but in another sense it is, because it is the spirit on a lower octave. Matter, therefore, is a mode of motion of spirit. This they have failed to see and in failing to see this, they have undertaken to deny its existence all the way through. The true view is that it does not exist as matter, but as the Maya of Spirit. Failing to recognize this differentiation of spirit, the Christian Scientists do not deal with it in the proper manner. The true method is to recognize the relation of spirit to matter, and conform in diet and outward habits and everything of the kind to the highest rules of hygiene, at the same time keeping the mind fixed in itself, thinking upon reality, and there can be no higher reality than the recognition that all things are emanations from God.

48

This is the supreme reality, and if the body be recognized as being a part of the universe which has emanated from God, as being, therefore, a creation of God and so, brought into harmony with all those things, the effect will be just as good from the point of view of Immortal Mind and there will be much less rubbish for Immortal Mind to clear away than what exists under present system.

Christian Science is, therefore, the erroneous outgrowth of an incomplete classification of nature. A deeper classification will ultimately express itself in a more perfect state of health. This is a modern version of the old drastic doctrine that matter is essentially evil; that it is not God created.

Matter is just as much a product of God as Spirit is. Of course, it is on a lower octave, but still it is a projection of God. The errors of mortal mind are the thinking of the human mind. Matter obeys the laws of God; man does not; therefore, the cause of sickness is not matter, but erroneous human thought. Let man obey the material laws; let him conform to nature in material things, and in his thinking conform to the absolute reason, to the Divine promptings, and then perfect health will express itself.

We see, therefore, that Christian Science is not perfect in its classification. With the great truth which it announces, which relates to mortal and Immortal Mind, it still fails to recognize the fundamental principle of the unity of nature, both spiritual and material. It discards matter in its classification, and thus propagates erroneous conceptions. This philosophy, which is ideal but not absolutely correct, must necessarily establish pictures of the same order in the mind of the patient, which will direct the vibratory forces and therefore, it must lead to a disordered, deranged state of mind. It does not enthrone Immortal Mind completely, but there is a distortion, a mixed consciousness, which expresses itself in and through the harmony and also through the inharmony; it is a state of confusion, chaotic and Cosmic, the Immortal and Mortal Mind mixed. It is for this reason that Christian Scientists very often get their conceptions mixed and their systems become out of order. Diseases grow up in spite of them because their system of thinking, their system of philosophy is not altogether correct. If they would purge out this incorrect conception and bring all their thinking into harmony with the Divine Mind, with the Immortal Mind, they would be able to entirely eliminate those pictures which express themselves in vibrations of disease, but owing to this distorted condition they do not always yield the best results.

It is in order to maintain their own Cosmos, to prevent any discordant influence, that they condemn the idea of reading any literature other than that of Christian Science. They oppose the idea of introducing other ideas which can establish conceptions out of harmony

49

with their own view; that is, out of harmony with those principles which they assume to be the realities of Immortal Mind and this is, from that point of view, perfectly correct. One's mind should be built up exclusively of truth, of the expressions of Immortal Mind if he would expect to have the influence of Immortal Mind manifested in his being.

However, Christian Scientists make the mistake of assuming that their teachings always manifest the perfection of Immortal Mind. This is owing to the fact that they have accepted certain abstract principles as being the dictate of Immortal Mind. These principles they have not fully tested, and in fact, many of them are emanations of mortal mind, and the application which is made of them by Scientists is invariably an off shoot of the Mortal Mind, consequently they cannot accomplish the work which they have in view.

But an ultimate Christian Science must be evolved, which will present nothing but the thoughts of Immortal Mind. By establishing these in the consciousness of the patient, by building up his mind with those thoughts of Immortal Mind and thus by establishing nothing but the Immortal pictures within, the vibrations naturally flowing from those pictures will determine the vibrations of the patient's entire Aura, consequently his inner principles will move in harmony with the absolute and eternal principles. Universal harmony must then be established throughout the entire system, and universal harmony must result in perfect health.

The difficulty in Christian Science is, therefore, not in any error in its fundamental principles with which it starts out, but in their limitations and the consequent erroneous applications which are made of those principles, which lead unto great difficulty in mankind's reaching Immortal Mind and bringing those universal abstractions into practical operation. Christian Science is perfect, but Christian Scientists are woefully imperfect. Because they do not embody and comprehend the fullness of Christian Science, they fall far short of realizing the results at which they aim.

L E S S O N
O N
C H R O M O P A T H Y

Remember what we have so often said, that form, sound and color
are inseparably connected with all vibratory activities. Whenever
energy is vibrating to a certain rate, that is, a certain rapidity or
a certain rhythm, those vibrations assume a form which is the result of
this rate; a definite geometrical figure which is the inevitable and
natural result of that particular rate of vibration. It also produces
a definite sound representing that particular rate of vibration. It
not only reproduces that sound, however, but it also assumes a certain
color. But it isn't our purpose to go into details in regard to esoteric
meanings of color, as that is very thoroughly dealt with in the 10th
lesson of our course in Motion and Number. We will simply deal with
them in relation to their therapeutic value.

The color of any subject is due to rhythm; it is the expression
in the line of color of the vibratory rate of that object — of the
energy composing it. The result is that whenever you see the color of
an object you are able to recognize the rate of vibration of that object, if you understand it. But that is not all, because color, form
and sound is the threefold manifestation of the one and self same state
of vibration; it follows, therefore, that if you form in mind a picture of a certain color, by the mere mental visualization upon a certain color you will, therefore, form the picture which will set up the
rate of vibration which corresponds to that color. In a word, by visualizing upon either the color, form or sound, by making this mental
picture upon your mind, the forces of your aura, will cause this vibration to be set up which will give expression to that form, color
or sound; and visualizing upon the attributes of a given rhythm will
tend to the establishment of that particular rhythm within the human
organism. As a result you may visualize upon the form, color or sound
and you will set up in your aura the rhythm which corresponds to it.

You can understand that as the only difference between health

and disease is difference in the state of vibration, it therefore, follows logically that any method, no matter what it may be, that will lead
into the establishment of the proper vibratory rates, states or conditions within the aura will for that reason be beneficial in the
highest degree.

Because color is related to certain states of vibration, meditation upon a certain color, the formation of a mental picture upon that
color, will have the tendency of establishing the rate of vibration
which corresponds to that color. The thing that we want to do above
everything else is to establish that rate of vibration. What we want to
do in this lesson is to ascertain the vibrations and effects in relation
to health of certain colors, and ascertain how, by meditating upon
these colors, in making a mental picture of them, the rate of vibration
may be established. This is merely the healing of disease through the
effect of color.

Let us begin with the various states of the various colors, and
try to ascertain their activity. We will take, to begin with, the
physical color, the color of the Etheric Double. This is Pink, or more
properly speaking, the color of a fresh blown peach blossom. Spleen
troubles are really disorders of the Etheric Double, invariably.
The Spleen is the organ through which the Double circulates; it circulates just as the blood circulates through the heart. Suppose there
is some disorder of the Spleen or disorder of the Etheric Double. You
want to stimulate the Etheric Double, to build up the Spleen, to give it
strength, you must increase the strength and power of the Etheric vibration. There are various methods of doing that. We are now studying
Chromopathy. You should, therefore, be there weakness of the Etheric
Double, wear PINK. There should be as much pink in the room as possible,
or fresh blown peach blossoms for a bouquet in the room. Pink should
be kept everlastingly before the eye of the patient, so that he will
see pink, and when he sees this it will thus keep a picture of it in the
mind. That picture will give expression to the vibratory rhythm corresponding to pink.

A patient was suffering from a kind of physical weakness and
she used this color. She had a pink dress made and had the most wonderful results from it — because it helped to establish this pink color
before her mind, it set up the vibration corresponding to it.

If you have a patient suffering from physical weakness, if the
Etheric principle is deteriorating, you want to increase that, you want
to build it up, working to that end, to that realization, we must go to
work and use everything that will call out the expression of that principle. If there is any spleen trouble (no matter what it is) the
chromopathic cure is PINK.

This is simply a matter of mental picturing and the picturing
of PINK will always produce the true condition for treating the Etheric

Double.

Suppose you have a patient with low vitality, his vital force is very low; we must of necessity, above everything else, remember the color of Prana. The vital force is Rose, and it is the only part of the Aura which is rose color. For this reason, instead of using other methods, simply establish in the mind of your patient a picture of ROSE color, and keep it perpetually before his mind, where he will always see it, and always realize that rose color. This will give him the rhythm of life from his seeing it. You should keep a bouquet of roses in the room where the patient is all the time. Encourage patient to wear roses as much as possible, have the room papered in rose color. If there is a rug of roses in the room, so much the better. Rose colored quilts, rose colored garments, in fact, any method which will establish or keep a picture of rose color in his mind will prove itself effective, will stimulate vital powers and vitality.

If patient's emotions are weak and you find it necessary to stimulate the circulation, stimulate the heart, which is under the control of the Astral Body, if you want to fill him with hope, optimism, to quicken all things emotional in the proper manner — use BLUE in the same way. It depends upon the degree of activity as to the kind of blue you should use. VIOLET, owing to its high rate of vibration, I have found the most powerful to stimulate an intense vibration of the Astral Body; to stimulate those activities in very high degree use VIOLET.

Whatever it be you employ those colors according to the condition you want to produce, if you want to produce a kind of spiritual effect, or emotional, and feel that patient really requires it, you should use a pale azure blue; if you would have spiritual emotion, use LAVENDER.

RED is the positive masculine color, — no matter what it may be, Red is the positive color and the masculine color, the color of the Will; and it matters not with what it is combined, it aids the volitional positive will. If you find a patient with a weakened will use RED for this purpose in the same way you would other colors. PURPLE which is a combination of RED and BLUE, is, therefore, the positive Will applied to emotion.

YELLOW is the color of intellect, it is the intellectual color. If you want to stimulate intellect, if you think the person needs intellectual activity, use YELLOW. If you want to stimulate intellect in connection with positive will, use ORANGE, in the same way, which likewise stimulates intuition. To stimulate pure reason GOLD may be used.

If you want to stimulate spiritual activity, if you feel the spiritual diseased — because he is either too material and has not sufficient spirituality, or is not sufficiently near the ideal (and patients have diseases where there is no apparent physical cause) if

53

you want to overcome this state use WHITE, which governs the vibration of the Spirit. But if you want to approach toward the material, don't want to get too far from material things, want to establish a connection between the spiritual and the material use GRAY, which is a mixture of black and white — as black mixes with white, so will be the proportion.

Whatever the influence you wish to establish, you simply use the color that corresponds to it.

Suppose you want to produce an active condition. You have a patient who is suffering from indisposition, there isn't anything the matter with him, but he hasn't energy to do anything, has a severe case of indisposition, apply GREEN. GREEN will establish rhythm, the vibration, which will prompt the person to action. GREEN stimulates in the direction of action. GREEN should not be used unless the person needs some stimulation to their activity.

BROWN is not advisable. It has a detrimental effect all the way through. BLACK is always decidedly detrimental — it being the color of DEATH, the color which governs the rhythm of death. Whenever a patient is sick, get rid of all the black in the room; don't ever wear anything black. Get rid of all the BLACK; don't allow anything BLACK in the place, and according to the condition of the patient, regulate the color of everything that comes into contact with him.

It is very important to regulate the rate of vibration. A nervous patient should never have anything of livid GREEN in the room. SCARLET will stimulate anger. CRIMSON is a very good color, it being the color of affection. GREEN is the best of all colors for stimulating action, and will be found beneficial in many respects. Some of the GRAY colors are not good, as they approach almost to the death color themselves. LEAD color is never advisable for the sick person; it is the color of Saturn, and that is the same as BLACK. Those colors should be left entirely out. LAVENDER is the most spiritual of all emotional colors; therefore, it produces the most spiritual emotion; wherever spiritual emotions are desirable use LAVENDER.

The principles of Chromopathy are simple. Use those colors which will bring the proper mental picture in the mind of the patient, and therefore, the mental rhythm which will be the outward picture of that picture. In adapting it to therapeutics we have to bear these rules and regulations in mind and use them accordingly. But if the proper color is employed it will have the most wonderful effect for producing that picture, and will therefore, act upon the state of physical health.

L E S S O N
O N
H E R M E T I C   M E D I C I N E

The Hermetic System of Therapeutics is best represented in the works of Paracelsus. There we have the clearest presentation that has ever been given of the system.

The principles of the Hermetic System are, the Law of Correspondence, the Law of Opposites, and strange as it may seem, these principles are at the foundation of modern medicine. The Doctrine of Similarities is the theory that there are certain diseased conditions which must be excited and driven out of the system. It was the belief in this principle which led Samuel Hahnemann to the formation of his Homeopathic System, namely any drug, for instance that will cause the same effect in a well man that is manifested in a certain sickness, a drug that will cause the symptoms of a disease, will cure the disease, and he assumes that it will do this because it will have the effect of stimulating that condition, awakening it into activity so that it will be driven out of the system, will purge it out by means of the awakening of that influence. Thus, the same principles which are manifested in a disease will help drive it out. The Law of Similarities is, therefore, made use of as a means of eliminating the condition.

The system on which the Tegular School is based, is the Law of Contraries, the view that the disease is due to a preponderance of a certain element and so the patient must be given the other element, and right here is recognized the Law of Opposites; give the other element to restore the equilibrium, and in this way overcome that evil tendency.

If Paracelsus had any of the spirit of revenge in his nature and if he could be conscious of the present state of the medical world, he would certainly be satisfied. His revenge has been complete. He has been denounced as a charletan, a mountebank and everything of the kind by all schools of medicine, and yet there is not a single school that is not literally following some of the axioms of his system. The regulars in their doctrine of giving the opposite, of overcoming the disease, are literally following one of his doctrines, and the Homeopathic School follows another law, the Law of Similars; the Eclectics, in their system of specific medication are following out his theory that the system requires certain elements and to supply these elements would establish health, specific medication being founded upon the assumption that the system is in need of certain elements and because of that need, because it is suffering from the lack of those elements, this pathological condition is established.

The works of Paracelsus today rule the System of Medicine from the Regulars to the Christian Scientists; they are all following in his footsteps.

Now, inasmuch as there is force enough in his system to dominate all these antagonistic schools, it becomes of the greatest importance that we should study those laws carefully and see just what is employed in them. The fundamental principle of his school is recognition of two principles, what we now term Electricity and Magnetism. These two principles are operative in all life in all nature. Everything that exists is but the manifestation of these two principles. When one of these principles is too prominent in the system, the application of the other principle will neutralize it and thus restore equilibrium, and this is the use of the Law of Opposites; we produce an effect opposite to that which is present; the system is under certain influences, is dominated by certain forces; we go to work and restore equilibrium. Thus we employ the Law of Opposites. Now, any method that will establish the other pole in the ascendency, will bring about relief. Sometimes it is not sufficient to put in the opposite principle, but there is an effect of this principle that must be driven out; that is to say, there has been formed a substance in the system which must lead to disease. This must be eliminated. To do this it becomes necessary to employ the Law of Similarities and by establishing this condition in a high degree, we drive out the influence, forcing it out of the system.

This Law of Correspondence is the foundation of the practical application of the system, namely, everything that is in you is in everything else. Man and every part of the Universe is a microcosm of the whole. Whatever is wanting in you is present in a small degree. In order to overcome the condition we must establish a greater percentage of this minimum principle. To do this Paracelsus resorted to remedies which contained a large quantity of this minimum principle, and it was for this reason that he made use of remedies. It should also be borne in mind that he recognized that any influence which is brought to bear upon a principle contained in a healing agent, will impart the same influence to man, will continue to act in that way when it is contained in the system, because every principle of this agent is contained in man also. Now, an effect accomplished in the remedy will reproduce itself in man. This is his doctrine and it is also preeminently the doctrine of the Spirit of the Drug. He does not pay any attention to the crude drug, to the body of the drug, but it is the spirit of the drug that is of vital importance to him. No drug is used merely with reference to its physical effect. It is resorted to because of its finer principles and those finer principles are not just what the crude drug would lead one to believe.

Hermetic Chemistry is, therefore, altogether different from ordinary physical chemistry. The influence of drugs is largely drawn from the seven principles of nature, as represented by the seven planets of the Old Alchemists, that is the Sun and Moon, Saturn, Jupiter, Mars, Venus and Mercury. The Sun represents the principle of gold and also the masculine principle of nature, and this gold must not be understood as simply metallic gold, it is in one sense, the spiritual principle. The Moon is really the Spirit of Silver, the Soul Spirit and also the magnetic principle and all the others are the result of the union of the Sun and the Moon. Venus is the Spirit of Copper — Mars of Iron, — Mercury of Mercury or Quicksilver, — Jupiter of Tin and Saturn of Lead. Now in order to get those influences he does not give metallic lead; that is the great mistake so many people have made in studying Paracelsus; they have supposed he meant those metals, but he means principles of nature. Now, according to Paracelsus, there are certain plants which embody those principles, also, — the same plants under certain planetary aspects will embody those principles.

Paracelsus, therefore, considers medicine worthless unless the herbs are gathered with reference to certain principles, certain planetary conjunctions, etc. It is the principles that he acts upon. This department more properly belongs under the head of Astrological Medicine, but bear in mind that Hermetic Medicine deals with Cosmic forces and regards the diseases of the body as being the effects of disastrous combinations of those Cosmic forces. It also regards them as being spiritual influences acting upon the physical nature. By establishing conditions in the finer principles of man's organism we cause them to descend to the physical body.

Each principle being an exact duplicate of the other, according to Paracelsus, if you can establish a certain state in the Etheric Double you will, by reason of that fact, cause that state to be established in the gross physical body; consequently he endeavors to establish conditions in the Etheric Principle, and he really treated disease in this way.

But Paracelsus also makes use of the doctrine of Mumia through which it is possible to establish the same condition in the Etheric Double of the patient that you establish in the ether contained within the Mumia. This merges on the realm of Magic, the doctrine of Mumia being that an effect produced in the mumia or ether of a patient when

57

separated from his body, will produce the same effect in the ether contained within the body, and it has been verified to a high degree by modern experiments. It has been found that shortly after amputation of a leg, the amputated leg had been removed to another room and pins thrust into it; the patient felt the pain, literally cried out with pain, complaining every time the pins were thrust in. Again when the dismembered limb was placed very near a fire so that it was very warm, the man felt the heat and complained about it.

There was one case where a man's leg was cut off and the leg nailed up in a coffin and buried. The man kept kicking and complaining that they had driven a nail into his leg and he felt it. He kept on until finally they took the coffin up, opened it and sure enough, found that in nailing up the box a nail had been driven into the leg. They took the nail out, put the leg back into the box, nailed it up properly and again buried it and the patient had no more trouble. Another man complained after his leg had been cut off and buried that they had his toes crossed and he kept on complaining until they actually had to dig up and straighten the toes before the patient could get any comfort.

There have been quite a number of cases of this kind, which show conclusively that there is a consciousness between a leg severed from a man, and the man and that such consciousness continues for some time. This is a manifestation of the doctrine that a connection is maintained between the Etheric Principle contained in a leg or any other part of the body, after it has been removed from the body, and the Etheric Double within the body. Thus a physical amputation does not sever the etheric principle, it is still One and what it senses, the man can sense.

This principle of Mumia has been made use of by sorcerers from time immemorial. They have always resorted to it as a means of accomplishing their ends. Paracelsus proposed to use it as a means unto the relief of suffering humanity. If an injury imparted to the mumia of a person will injure the Etheric Double of the patient, and therefore, react upon his body, so will a benefit conferred upon the mumia result in a benefit to the Etheric Double and, therefore, to the gross physical body, so Paracelsus applied this principle and the results are wonderful. He treated blood poison, for instance, by having a certain quantity of blood taken from the man's veins and taken into a vessel. This poison blood, after being removed from the patient's veins, he treats and when he has purified and has cured that blood, the blood in the patient's veins will be found to be pure. In this way he treats blood poison, through the Law of Correspondences, or the Law of Sympathies as we term it. In the same way he cures a headache, by treating a lock of hair cut from the man's head, he cures the man. He cured more cases of headache and blood poison than any of the other doctors. Again we find him treating dog bites by treating the dog, not the man.

58

He cured snake bites, when it was possible to capture the snake, by making the snake take the medicine, and in this way destroying the poison in the snake and, by the Law of Correspondences it destroyed the poison in the patient. He treated a wound not by putting medicine in the wound, not by disinfecting the wound, but by disinfecting the weapon.

Now, how is this accomplished? Obviously the etheric principle of the patient is on the weapon to a certain extent and by acting upon this, he acts upon the patient. Also the etheric principle of the weapon has entered into that of the patient and disturbance has taken place, so by this connection he is able to accomplish the change. Paracelsus treated the garments of people, and everything of that kind, as a means unto the curing of disease in the patients, and the entire rationale of this system is the connection which takes place in the mumia and through sympathy, in the Etheric Double of the patient; if you can accomplish this, you can accomplish the cure. Mumia is contained in everything that has been severed from the body of the patient or in any way removed from his body, and contains the Etheric Principle. The hair, the teeth, the skin, any part of the body, the bones, everything of that kind of a dead man contain his mumia and by removing this mumia we can get rid of the disease.

Also, sometimes methods are resorted to which are very unjust, very unfair. Albertus Magnus recognizing the same principle, resorted to the practice of taking the mumia of a sick person and fixing it up in a bundle and then laying the bundle down where some one could pick it up and open it. The result would be the mumia would come in contact with that person's etheric principle and if he were at all negative, would establish the disease and when he contracted the disease it would leave the Etheric Principle of the patient, going to this second party, this poisonous condition could come to him. This, of course, is not a legitimate application of the doctrine, yet such application has been made by quite a number.

Paracelsus places the greatest emphasis upon the Law of Sympathies and upon those methods which make use of correspondences. He says, for instance, that he has learned from the professors and with this conception, of course, he favors very highly those methods which make use of correspondences. Remember the fundamental principle in this; any influence set in operation within the Etheric Double will influence the physical body. The healing art is, therefore, the art of establishing proper vibratory conditions and vibratory influences within the Etheric Double and every part of Mumia taken from the body of the patient corresponds to and is one with the Etheric Principle contained within the double. Any effect produced in the mumia will act upon the ether in the double and thus will give rise to a corresponding effect; will become a cause in the work.

To impart a vibration to the mumia will, therefore, through sympathy, impart the same vibration to the Etheric Double, therefore, medicines given to blood taken from your veins or to a lock of hair cut from your head, to the parings of your nails, to your old clothes, or anything of that kind, to the water in which you have bathed, to the excretory eliminations of the body will have precisely the same effect as taking the medicine internally will have. In fact, it will act much more directly, because in this method you impart it to the etheric principle, whereas by taking it internally it has to go through the physical body. It is less harmful and more effective, therefore, to medicate the mumia, than to medicate the physical body direct.

Medicines owe their healing efficacy to the principles contained within them, and it is, therefore, that we should have reference to the seven healing potencies of Nature, namely, Sol, Luna, Mercury, Venus, Mars, Jupiter and Saturn, and there are various ways by which this is to be accomplished; whichever method will yield the best results is to be resorted to.

Disease and Health are shown by Paracelsus to be relative conditions and to be governed by the Law of Correspondences, the Law of Sympathies and Antipathies, the Law of Opposites. It is the application of those principles that is at the foundation of the Hermetic Healing Art.

Some other features of this system do not seem to be quite so logical as even this. For instance, Paracelsus claims that certain things, certain flowers, and herbs, owe their healing potency to the fact that they are Sun colored; that they manifest the color of the Sun; that it is not because of their chemical colors, but because of their personal appearance, their color, that they exercise their healing influence, but if we realize that color itself is the effect of vibration, the effect of certain specific rates of vibration, then it will be seen that Paracelsus is not so very far wrong after all. Anything is Sun-Color because it has the solar vibrations, therefore, the Aura of anything Sun-Colored will bring the Solar vibration. Blackness is due to the influence of Saturn, not of course, to the influence of the planet Saturn, specifically, but to the Saturnine force, that force, that principle which is the keynote of the Planet Saturn. Chemicals which are black, therefore, owe their blackness to their Saturnine principle and consequently, will exercise Saturnistic influence.

The Solar color of Gold and everything of that kind owes its color to the Solarian principle and, therefore, will impart that vibration to the system.

White is due to the Lunar principle and will impart that lunar vibration to the system.

Red is due to the Martian principle and will impart that vibration.

Thus we see when Paracelsus divides herbs in reference to their color into different chemical groups, he has really found the fundamental cause of all chemical differentiation and instead of this being silly, it is really true, it is fundamental, it is exact science.

Again he assumes that certain things will benefit the heart, owing to their heart shape; that because they are shaped like the heart they exercise a beneficial effect on the heart and you will see that he is right, when you realize that all form is the effect of vibratory influence, that the form is evolved as a result of definite rates of vibration in the ether; that every geometrical figure owes its specific shape to the vibration of the forces. It will, therefore, be seen that heart-shaped flowers, leaves, and everything of the kind are in that shape because they have that specific rate of vibration. The heart is a symbol, representing the Desire Principle. It is formed by the activity of certain forces, consequently when heart-shaped leaves and flowers are used as medicine, they transmit to the Astral Body those Desire vibrations and stimulate it. The Astral is thus effected and because it is effected, it strengthens the heart, which is its physical organ. Thus the use of heart-shaped flowers and leaves as medicines to stimulate the heart, instead of being superstition, is the most fundamental physics. It is the bringing to bear the deepest principle of transcendental physics, upon the treatment of the body.

The Law of Correspondences is at the foundation of all existence, the Law of Sympathy and Antipathy is the cause of all centrifugal and centripetal force and as all manifestation is the expression of those two forces, everything operates through it. Therefore, Paracelsus, the prince of physicians, was in reality employing the deepest principles of nature in the healing of the body. By healing the Etheric Double, thus acting upon the Body, he is realizing the constitution of man and acting through it. When he finds a weakness in a certain organ, he finds that principle in man's Aura which functions through it, he then treats the principle and by reflex action, the organ. He would, therefore, treat the spleen by treating the Etheric Double; the Solar Plexus and the entire sympathetic nervous system, not by treating the nerves at all, but by treating the Prana; he would treat the heart by treating the Astral Body; the brain he would treat, not by treating the physical organ, but by treating the mind. He would treat the Pineal Gland by interesting the soul, etc., etc., all the way through he would find the subtile principle which operates through a given organ and then stimulate that to produce the proper effects.

The methods of Paracelsus are, therefore, absolute and exact science applied to the treatment of the body, through the Constitution of Man. Instead of being superstition and charlatanry they are the philosophy of philosophies, the only scientific medicine, including Astrological Medicine (which is really another branch of Hermetic Med-

61

icine).

We may say that Hermetic Medicine embraces three branches, that which we have included under this head, — second Astrological Medicine, and third, what might be termed Magnetic or Sacramental Healing, the Blessing of articles, etc., the use of Holy Water, oil-blessed articles and everything of that kind.

These three branches include one of the greatest features of the healing Art. Hermetic Medicine in its threefold aspect, really gives us the best part in fact, the only fundamental efficacy of Materia Medica.

LESSON
ON
ASTROLOGICAL MEDICINE

The foundation of the second division of Hermetic Medicine, Astrological Medicine, is in the influence emanating from the Sun, the Moon, the Planets and the different Signs of the Zodiac. There are in the different Signs of the Zodiac influences that act upon different parts of the body. Each sign corresponds to a certain region and will stimulate that region in the body, consequently there are organic and functional diseases that are due to affliction by the Zodiacal Signs and Planets, each part of the body being stimulated by the activity of that particular Sign or Planet, powerful state of health will grow out of the stimulation of the faculty when the stimulation is only normal, but when it reaches an abnormal degree the equilibrium is overturned and functional disturbance takes place, just the same as the disturbance when the amount of Prana going to a nerve center has been more than that nerve center could conveniently deal with.

Again, if one part of the body is over stimulated it may lead to the under stimulation or starving of the opposite part of the body; consequently all those disturbances partaking of the nature of functional diseases may grow out of the over stimulation of certain parts of the body by Zodiacal influence.

It should also be borne in mind that at the time the Sign of one's nativity is active, its influence is more than twice as great as the influence of any other sign would be; that is, one born under the sign Aries will suffer twice as much from affliction of Aries as one born under any other Sign, as he already has a powerful development of the Aries quality. The head is naturally sensitive and naturally active owing to that influence. Now, an abnormal development or activity coming from over stimulation from Aries will create a still greater disturbance than it would in one in whom the equilibrium was better maintained. You should realize, therefore, that the coincidence of the Birth Sign with the bodily sign must always give a much greater degree of stimulation and when

63

this coincides also with the same moon sign, it is then a tremendous force.

A number of diseases are caused by infliction from the Zodiacal influence as well as from the planetary influences and for this reason it will be found of great utility to have the Zodiacal and Planetary influences applied as therapeutic agents. It should be borne in mind that the Laws of Sympathy and Antipathy both operate in this case and sometimes it is necessary to resort to the Law of Opposites, by opposing a contrary influence to counteract the over stimulation and thus restore the equilibrium. At other times it is found advantageous to employ the Law of Similarities and rather increase the operation of that principle which is causing the disturbance so as to purge out certain influences.

As a general rule where there are poisons it is best to increase the disturbance so as to drive them out, but where it is simply a functional trouble, then it is best to use the Law of Opposites and restore the equilibrium.

The method of treatment under consideration is, therefore, the application of Zodiacal and Planetary influences as therapeutic agents.

Well, the question then naturally comes up, how are they to be employed as therapeutic agents? How are we to get those influences so that we can use them? They are secured through certain plants, minerals, etc. Drugs, in fact, embody these principles. They have their nativities the same as people have, being under the influence of the different signs of the Zodiac and the different planets — having embodied those influences and will transmit them to the patient, when they are taken. Drugs when used in this way, become the channels for transmitting healing virtues from the Signs of the Zodiac and the different Planets, to the body.

There are certain classes of plants, spices, etc., which influence different parts of the body because they have those Zodiacal and Planetary influences. Then there are other classes of plants that are under the influence of a certain Sign and carry that chemical force.

Again, it will be found that under the different Signs of the Zodiac and the different planetary influences, all plants gathered at such times will communicate this influence. Before going into this matter it will be found advantageous to first ascertain the different parts of the body that the Signs control and consequently, the diseases likely to come from those signs. Remember, these diseases are due to the over stimulation or affliction of those different parts of the body. Aries rules the head; its influence, therefore, gives stimulation to the brain, and the cerebellum, the medulla oblongata, in fact, all the organs of the brain, and to the cerebro-spinal nervous system, the special senses, and governs, consequently, the circulation of the life force or nervous energy. Any disease due to over stimulation of any of those functions will be due to the affliction of Aries. Troubles of the eyes, the hearing, taste, touch, smell, nervousness, apoplexy, headaches, and all diseases of that type, when not caused by a weakened condition, are due to affliction. But if any of those senses are weak, if there be a case of locomotor ataxia or epilepsy, if it be a case of low vitality, if the nerve force is not strong enough, or if there be failing memory, weak mindedness, then the condition is due to a lack of the influence of Aries. All those afflictions controlled by Aries manifest themselves in weakness when there is a lack of this influence, and in over stimulation, over activity when there is too much of the Aries influence.

In these negative states it will be found, therefore, advantageous to give Aries, and by giving Aries we mean to give those medicines under the influence of Aries, which will act as channels for the communication of that influence, and if there be an over stimulation it will be found advantageous to use something that will exercise the corresponding influence, such, for instance, as are under the Sign of Pisces, so as to change the influence altogether, and this is on the same principle as the old medical practice of putting a mustard plaster on the stomach to draw inflammation from the brain. The point is to use some other influence, that will exercise just the reverse influence, or, it will be found advantageous to take the other extreme; for instance, those under the Sign Libra which will counterbalance it, drawing the influence down. Those medicines governed by Libra are, therefore, better than the ones governed by any other sign, as modifiers of the Aries influence.

The herb particularly under the influence of Aries is the Sage, and in order to stimulate the influence of Aries there is nothing so advantageous as the use of sage. The practice of the old women in using sage tea is, therefore, really an application of the principle of Aries. If you want to make use of incense, Myrrh is the greatest stimulus for Aries in the world. Where the Aries influence is weak, in all those diseases growing out of that condition, there is nothing so advantageous as burning, say a teaspoonful of Myrrh in a brazier, daily. It will do more good for such diseases than all the medicine in the world, ordinarily employed. However, in using myrrh, only that which is brought from Arabia, Persia or India should be employed, and the finest quality, as it has a much stronger force than the ordinary myrrh.

TAURUS governs the neck and throat. It, therefore, is the influence required in tonsilitis, catarrh, sore throat, croup and all troubles of that description — in all troubles of the neck and throat. When catarrh, croup, tonsilitis, etc., are efforts on the part of nature to purge out inflammation, they are, therefore, due to the influence of Taurus, but as the inflammation ought to be gotten rid of as the poison should be eliminated, the way to cure them is not to try to counterbalance, but to over stimulate them, to continue to add to the stimulation in order to get rid of the poison. Vervain is the plant peculiarly under the influence of Taurus, and will exercise this influence. Pimpernel is the fumigation to be used.

GEMINI governs the shoulders, arms, chest, consequently all troubles of the arms and hands, consumption, bronchitis and all troubles of the chest - everything of that kind, are due to the influence of Gemini. If there is a weakness in these regions it is because the influence of Gemini is wanting; if the trouble is due to over activity it indicates over stimulation; consequently, if you want to restore equilibrium by placing some other influence there, you should then use those influences, or those medicines which are influenced by Sagittarius. But if you want to increase the influence of Gemini, then, use as a fumigation Mastic, and as the herb, the Vervain is the natural medicine for all chest troubles where you wish to stimulate.

CANCER rules the breasts, mammary glands, stomach and diseases resulting from over stimulation are due to too much of the influence of Cancer and should be counterbalanced by the influence of Capricorn.

LEO governs the heart. All palpitation of the heart, every disease of the heart infection due to over stimulation, is due to too much of the influence of Leo and should be counterbalanced by the influence of Aquarius. If the trouble be a weakness of the heart, however, (and that means, also the entire circulation), if there be atrophy or fatty degeneration of the heart, anything wrong with the heart action, also with the arteries and veins, the circulatory system generally, if weak, should be stimulated by the stimulation of Leo. Sowbread is the medicine and Frankincense the spice for the fumigation.

VIRGO governs the stomach, the solar plexus and therefore, the sympathetic nervous system, nutrition and nourishment of the body and where this is weak it should be stimulated by the influence of Virgo. Where it is excessive it may be balanced by the influence of Pisces. The fumigation for Virgo is Sanders and the herb is Calamint.

LIBRA governs the umbilicus, the bowels and the digestive forces which act within the bowels, such as the pancreas, the liver as it generates bile, and the kidneys, the eliminative principles and everything connected with that part of the body, and also governs that section of the entire body corresponding; therefore, the lumbar region, and where those parts of the body are weak, its affinities should be given. Where they are over stimulated the influence of Aries should be resorted to. The affinity of Libra is the Mugwort and its fumigation is Galbanum.

SCORPIO governs the generative organs, the sacral plexus and all that part of the body. Sexual impotency and all weakness of the ovaries, fallopian tubes, the uterus — in fact all weaknesses of the sexual region and of the pelvis generally, is due to an insufficient stimulus from this sign, while venereal diseases, such as gonorrhoea, gleet, syphilis and other diseases of that type are due to its over stimulus, but there is a poison there which is being eliminated by the activity of Scorpio, consequently the cure for these troubles is the stimulation so that the poisons will be purged out. If we, therefore, continue to drive out the poison by continuing to stimulate the influence of Scorpio, we will succeed in accomplishing the cure. Scorpio is to be used for those diseases, but such diseases as nervousness, a dried up condition, a terribly spiteful character — those troubles, in fact growing out of unsatisfied sexual desire, are due to the over stimulus of Scorpio, and therefore, should be treated by the stimulation of Aries, and Taurus.

It is quite logical that sexual desire should be cured by stimulation of the head, that being the logical remedy for anything of that kind. The herb particularly embodying the principle of Scorpio is Scorpion grass, and the spice for the fumigation is Opopanax.

SAGITTARIUS governs the thighs, and all troubles of that region, whatever they may be, if they be weaknesses, should be treated by the stimulation of this influence, by the use of Pimpernel, and the fumigation is Lignum Aloes; while if it be over stimulated, it may be restrained by the influence of Gemini.

The knees are governed by CAPRICORN, and where a weakness is present should be treated with Dock and with the fumigation of Benjamin.

The legs are governed by AQUARIUS and all troubles in this region when weakness is evident, should be treated by a fumigation of Euphorbium, and where it is found necessary to restrain this influence we may employ Leo. In the case of tumors, or sore legs — anything of that nature, there is a poison which is trying to be eliminated, which is being driven out by the influence coming from Aquarius, which should be stimulated by more of the Aquarian influence. The herb for Aquarius is dragon's-wort.

PISCES governs the feet. All troubles of the feet should be treated by the stimulation of Pisces; this is true of all weakened conditions, such as chilblains and everything of that nature. Feet that have been frostbitten may be restored in this way. A case of gout should also be treated by the influence of Pisces. If it be found advisable to restrain the Pisces influence, then Virgo may be employed. The influence of Pisces may be secured through Hart's foot. Red Storax is the spice to be used for fumigation.

It should also be borne in mind that the planetary influences exercise a great therapeutic action.

MARS, being the same as Aries, governs the head and has practically the same influence on the body that the sign of Aries has.

VENUS is the same as Taurus; — MERCURY the same as Gemini and, therefore, should be used in the same way that the others would be used.

Before taking up the various planetary influences it will, perhaps, be well to look a little further into the different Zodiacal
medicines.

The influence of ARIES causes smallpox and fevers. Where animal
medicines are desired to be used, the oil extracted from the wolf will
be found to convey the same influence. Its plants are the briar,
holly, thistle, dock, fern, myrtle, mustard, onion, poppies, radish,
rhubarb and pepper. Part of these may be taken as food; the others
used as medicine. The wearing of the amethyst will also bring this
influence.

TAURUS may be secured by wearing agates and using beets, coltsfoot, columbine, daisies, dandelions, cresses, myrtle, phlox, mosses,
spinach.

The influence of GEMINI may be secured by wearing the beryl and
by using such plants as dog-grass, madder, woodbine, tansy and
yarrow.

The emerald will give the influence of Cancer and it should be
borne in mind that cancer governs the breasts, controls the mammary
glands, lactation and everything of that kind. Its influence may be
secured by eating cucumbers, squash, melons and all watery vegetables,
also by taking comfrey and fumigating with camphor.

LEO may be stimulated by wearing the ruby, by the use of
daffodil, dill, celandine, eye bright, fennel, St. John's wort,
lavender, poppy, marigold, mistletoe, parsley and pimpernel.

VIRGO will be attracted by wearing the jasper and by eating
endive, millet, privet, succory, scull cap, by eating wheat, barley,
oats and rye, as they are all under its influence.

LIBRA is attracted by the diamond; also by watercress, white
rose, strawberry, heartsease, palm, thyme and the pansy.

The influence of SCORPIO is secured by wearing the topaz and by
using the black thorn, horehound, pine, leeks and wormwood.

SAGITTARIUS is attracted by wearing the carbuncle and by using
agrimony, featherfew.

The influence of CAPRICORN is secured by wearing the chalcedony
and using the hemlock, henbane, holly, nightshade and black poppy.
This also is the house of Saturn and what applies to Saturn will apply
to this.

AQUARIUS, which is the house of Uranus, and therefore governed
by all those under the Uranic influence, is attracted by wearing the
sky-blue sapphire and using spikenard.

PISCES may be attracted by wearing the chrysolite, and as it is
the house of Neptune, sea weeds, ferns and mosses that grow in the
water.

The planetary influences should be adapted to the Signs to which they belong, and the Sun should be understood as being the masculine principle, while the Moon is the feminine. They are practically the same thing, though to a great extent, the lunar influence is similar to that of Uranus and the solar influence similar to that of Neptune. In the ancient days when they knew nothing about Uranus and Neptune, the Sun and Moon were used to represent the principles which we now represent by Uranus and Neptune.

The Solar influence may be secured by using such stones as the Eye of the Sun, the carbuncle, the chrysolite, the iris, the heliotrope and the hyacinth, the pyrophylus, the ruby and the auripigmentum, the wearing of these stones will attract the solar influence. The following named plants will also be found to give its influence; the marigold, the date-tree and therefore, the use of dates, the peony, the bay tree, cedar, pear tree, ash nut, mastic, zedoary, saffron, balsam, amber, musk, aloes, cinnamon, pepper, sweet marjoram.

The Lunar influence may be secured through the moonstone, the pearl, stalactite, beryl, aqua-marine and silver. Gold always gives the solar influence. By the use of such plants as the hyssop, rosemary, and olive, its influence may be secured.

It should be borne in mind that the same plant may embody two or three influences. Where it does, of course, in giving it to secure one, we must be sure that the other influence is not detrimental.

The influence of Saturn is secured by wearing onyx, using loadstone, and by the various preparations of lead, if taken as medicine or having lead ornaments. The plants embodying this principle are daffodils, dragon's-wort, mandrake opium, elderberry, black fig tree, and also black figs as a fruit, the cypress.

The influence of Jupiter may be secured by using the hyacinth, sapphire, emerald, green jasper and by wearing tin as a metal. The plants embodying this principle are the sea-green garden basil, mace, spike, mint, mastic, elecampane, daffodil, henbane, poplar, holly tree, poplar tree — therefore the use of potash, will be found advantageous, the hazel tree, also hazel nuts; service tree, and service berries; white fig tree and white figs as a diet, pear tree and pears as a diet, apple tree and the apple as food, the vine (that means the grapevine) plum tree, ash dog tree and the olive tree; olives also contain a certain amount of this principle, cereals of all kinds, raisins, sugar and almonds, pineapples, pistachio-nuts, rhubarb and storax. These will all be found to give this influence.

For Mars, the loadstone, the bloodstone and the jasper will be found beneficial. Iron and lead are the metals. The following plants will be found to give this influence: hellebore, garlic, euphorbium, radishes, anemone, laurel, wolf's-bane, cardis, nettle, crow-foot, onions, leeks, mustard seed.

The influence of Venus, which is the planet governing the neck

69

and throat, is secured by such stones as the beryl, chrysolite, emerald, sapphire and green jasper. The metals are silver, and brass or copper; silver because it is the feminine of magnetic metal and because the influence of Venus is much more magnetic than electric.

Venus not only influences the neck, however, but also the love principle and the sex desire, and therefore, has a great deal of influence on Scorpio as well as on Taurus. The plants that draw this influence are the violet, maidenhair, red sandalwood, sweet pea, the Rose of Lucifer, and the myrtle.

Mercury controls the breasts and arms and its influence may be secured also by the use of emeralds, and glass. The metals are quicksilver, and all such plants as the hazel, cress, the herb mercury, pimpernel, marjoram and parsley.

In a general way, everything that bears fruit embodies the influence of Jupiter; everything that bears flowers, flower-bearing herbs, and flowers of all kinds, embody the influence of Venus; all seed and bark, Mercury and all roots Saturn. All wood is from Mars, while all leaves are from the Moon.

If you want to lay out a diet for your patient, the Moon influence will be secured by the use of vegetables, while the influence of Saturn, by giving roots that grow under ground — Cereals will, to a great extent give the influence of Mercury. The use of all kinds of seeds and a diet of fruits will give the influence of Jupiter. Venus is secured by the use of flowers. The Japanese system of making salads from the petals of flowers gives a tremendous quantity of Venus influence.

The strongest planetary affinities, however, are from Saturn, the daffodil; from Jupiter, the henbane; from Mars, the ragwort; from the Sun, the knutgrass; from Venus, the vervain; from Mercury, the cinquefoil; from the Moon the goosefoot. Aries has asparagus; Scorpio the garden basil among its greatest forces.

Fumigation for the different planets may be used as follows: Pepperwort to secure the influence of Saturn; nutmeg for Jupiter; lignum aloes for Mars; mastic for the Sun; saffron for Venus; cinnamon for Mercury; and the Myrtle for the Moon. These influences will be found to manifest themselves sometimes in quite a number of different plants and also a number of different influences will be found in the same plant.

Likewise it will be found that the Sun's influence may be secured from almonds, angelica, camomile, celandine, centaury, corn hornwort, eyebright, heart trefoil, juniper, mistletoe, mustard, olive, pimpernel, rosemary, rice, meadow-rue, saffron, St. John's wort, St. Peter's wort, sundew, tormentil, turnsole, Viper's bugloss, vine and walnut.

The Lunar influence may be secured through adder's tongue, cabbage, colewort, caltrops, (water) chickweed, clary, cleavers coral-wort, cuckoo flowers, cucumbers, cress, daisy, dogtooth, Buck's-meat, iris, lettuce, lilies, loose-strife, mercury, moon-wort, mouse-ear, orpine, pearlwort, privet, pumpkin, purslain, rattlegrass, saxifrage (winter) stonecrop, trefoil, waterflag, wallflowers, (water) arrow-head, water cress, water lily, water violet, white poppy, white lily, white rose, whitlow grass, wild wallflower, wintergreen, willows.

The Mercurial influence may be secured through amara-dulcis, azaleas, calamint, carraway, wild carrots, coraline, cow parsnips, dill, elecampane, endive, fern, fennel, germander, hare's foot, hazel nut, horehound, hound's tongue, lavender, lily of the valley, liquorice, male fern, mandrake, maidenhair (white), maidenhair (golden), mulberry, myrtle, nailwort, olive spurge, oats, wild parsley, pellitory of the wall, southernwood, star-wort, scabious, smallage, valerian, winter savoury.

The Venusian influence for the neck may be secured through the use of alkanet, alehoof, alder tree, both black and common, arrack, archangel (wild and stinking) artichokes, beans, birch, bishop's-weed, bramble, blites, bugle, holly, burdock cherry, chestnut, (earth) chick-pease, cock's-head, columbines, coltsfoot, couchgrass, cowslip, cranesbill, cudweed, crabsclaw, crosswort, devil's-bit, dropwort, elder, featherfew, figwort, foxglove, groundsel, ground-ivy, gromel, goldenrod, gooseberry, herb Robert, kidney wort, ladies' bedstraw, ladies' mantle, little daisy, marshmallows, mercury, (dog) mercury (French), mints (various) mint-money-wort, motherwort, mugwort, orchis, parsley, pennyroyal, pennywort, peppermint, peach tree, pear tree, plums, poppy, privet, queen of the meadows, ragwort, rose (Damask), red cherries, sanicle, self-heal, soapwort, sorrel, sowthistle, strawberry, spignel, tansy, teasel, thyme, throatwort, vervain, violets, wheat, yarrow.

The influence of Mars for the head may be secured through all-heal, aloes, barberry, basil, box-tree, broom, briony, brooklime, butcher's broom, broomrape, carduus benedictus, civet, cresses (various) cotton-thistle, capers, catmint, coriander, dove's-foot, dragon's flaxweed, dyer's-weed, furzebush, gentian, hawthorne, honey-suckle, hops, horse-tongue, hedge hyssop, horseradish, leeks, madder, masterwort, mousetail, mustard, onions, pepperwort, pine, rocket, rhubarb, starthistle, slavin, tobacco, wormwood, wake robin, and also to a great extent by using wheat when the whole wheat grain is usually indicated.

The influence of Jupiter may be secured through agrimony, aniseed, asparagus, alexander, avens, balm, balsam, beet (white) betony, bilberry, borage, bloodwort, chervil, chestnut tree, cinque-foil, costmary, dandelion, dock, dog-grass, endive, fig tree, gilli-flowers, hart's tongue, hyssop, houseleek, jessamine, liverwort, lungwort, lime-wort, maple, myrrh, melitot, nailwort, oak, pinks,

(Wild), roses (red), sage, scurvy-grass, succory (wild), samphire, swallow-wort, thistle, thorn apple.

Saturn's influence, governing the knees is secured through the use of aconite, amaranthus, barley, barren-wort, beech-tree, beet (red), black hellebore, bluebottle, bifoil, birdsfoot, bistort, black-thorn, bucksthorn, plantain, clown's woundwort, comfrey, crosswort, flaxweed, fleawort, fumitory, gladwin, ground moss, goutwort, heart-ease, hawkweed, hemp, henbane, horsetail, holly, ivy, Jew's ear, knap-weed, knot-grass, mosses, medlar, navelwort, poplar, quince, rupture-wort, rushes, rye, service tree, spleenwort, sloes, sciatica-wort, Solomon's seal, tulsan, thistle.

It should also be borne in mind that at the time a certain planet is ruling the earth all the herbs are governed by that influence and take it on, so that they are all influenced by it. If you will, there-fore, gather your own medicines — botanic medicines and gather them at such time as they are under a certain influence, you will find they will have that influence. It is for this reason that medicines are so slightly to be relied upon when bought in a pharmacy, no attention hav-ing been paid to the planetary influence when they were gathered even to the day and hour as upon what the particular medicine is. The works on materia medica do not take into consideration to any degree whatever the time at which herbs are gathered, but it is absolutely necessary to do this in order to get valuable results.

```
L E S S O N

O N

M A G I C A L   H E A L I N G
```

By this term we mean the blessing of articles and thus communicating to them a magnetism which may be imparted to the body of the
patient and thus heal him.

The earliest instance we find of this is the case of Elijah
dropping his mantle to Elisha in order that he might receive a double
portion of his spirit. The mantle, having been thoroughly magnetized
by that Spirit when worn by Elijah had become a vehicle for the communication of that force to whoever put it on.

The next instance is the case of Elisha sending his servant to
lay his staff upon a person, that he might be healed. The staff had
become magnetized by being carried in the hand of Elisha and curing
was received by it.

Again we find in the New Testament several instances of persons
bringing aprons and other garments to St. Peter that he might touch
them and then they might be placed upon the sick person and thus heal.
All through the New Testament there is a distinct recognition of the
ability of a Saintly person of high development, a person with great
magnetic and spiritual power to so impart his power to the article that
when placed upon a patient it will impart the healing magnetism.

Previous to the New Testament time this was simply the use of
an article magnetized in a causal way, but in the New Testament time
we find the distinct practice of magnetizing articles for the express
purpose of healing.

Again we find that the practice was resorted to by the early
church for the purpose of imparting spiritual powers. The doctrine
of consubstantiation is perfectly true. The blessing of bread and
wine imparts to it a spiritual element which is neither bread nor wine
but when taken into the system it will fill one's spirit with that
spiritual force. The use of holy water in certain ceremonies is
another instance. By imparting the blessing to the water it becomes

magnetically charged, receives a certain principle and when used will communicate that influence to the inner principles of the being.

The entire Jewish religion, so far as its ritual is concerned, is built upon a recognition of this principle. Why does the Jew refuse to eat with unwashen hands? Simply because the ceremonial washing of the hands imparts a certain magnetic force which removes the influence which he takes on by reason of his contact with the world. Again, the use of clean water in certain ceremonies is a recognition of this principle. Clean water consisted of water containing a small quantity of the ashes of a red heifer without blemish, burned by the priest in sacrifice. This would impart ceremonial cleanliness. It was not simply a ceremony, however, it really drove out a great deal of unclean magnetic force, cleaning the system. It also imparted a spiritual influence. When the Jews change the dishes and everything, the cover, even going over the table with a hot iron, when they change from a dinner of dairy products, etc., to one of meat, it is for the same purpose. These ceremonies impart a changed magnetism.

We see again in India the recognition of the danger of contracting another's personal magnetism. For this reason high caste Brahmans always have nine feet square assigned to themselves in the floor, sit in the middle of it and never allow a person to cross the line. They will never shake hands with, will never touch one who is not of their own caste and not even then if they can possibly avoid it. The Brahman wants to protect himself from the magnetism of others and in this way he does it.

When the Guru sends forth the Chela, invested with the Brahmanic degree and carrying a rod in his hand which has been blessed by the Guru, the Chela is thus invested with the magnetic power of his Master. It abides in his rod and may be exercised in that way.

Many of the sacraments of the church were for the same purpose. Extreme unction and confirmation are for that purpose of imparting certain powers, certain spiritual forces to the spirit of the communicant.

The garments which one wears become charged with his magnetism and if another one puts them on, they will transmit that force. It is, therefore, very wrong for people to give their clothes to people who may be injured by their magnetism. One who is on a higher plane than you are should not wear your clothes or anything you have had on. You should not allow a person who is on a lower plane than you, to have your clothes and you then wear them again unless you intend to practice a little self sacrifice of a very high order. On the contrary — you should never under any consideration lend one of your garments to one who is your superior unless you intend to steal his magnetism and get rid of some of your own meanness. People are continually being

influenced in this way; the magnetic force is continually passing out
and exercising its influence. For this reason one should have different garments for different purposes. The Jewish custom of wearing
the prayer scarf at prayers and never putting it on at any other time,
is ideal. It is from a recognition of that magnetic principle, because
at the time of prayer his whole being is devotional; the devotional
atmosphere is all around him and at that time his prayer scarf is being
saturated with this magnetism of devotion, and when he puts it on again
it reacts upon him and thus stimulates the devotional side of his
being.

The custom of wearing a head covering at the synagogue is also
ceremonial; likewise the custom of wearing the kettle at the Passover
is ceremonial, inasmuch as it stimulates that feeling which he has
at that particular time, that being the most solemn of all the
festivals of the Jewish religion.

A person should have a certain costume to wear at church and
should never put it on at any other time. Likewise if he can afford
several, it will be found to be quite advantageous so that he may wear
different costumes at different services. The business suit should
never ever be worn at any other time because it is in that costume that
one transacts business with the world and the influence he gets at
that time, his thinking, etc., will influence his being at other times
if he continues to wear it. When he goes into society he should have a
suitable costume, which he should wear on no other occasion. The
custom of wearing the dress suit is most desirable inasmuch as no man
will ever be guilty of putting on a dress suit when he does not have
to put it on, consequently, the wearing of it on social occasions will
draw the bad vibrations of his associates and it will also become associated with the white lies that he tells on such occasions and as
soon as it is removed he will lay aside that personality. It should
consequently be sufficiently ridiculous that no man or woman will ever
put it on at a time when social usage does not require it. Then there
should be other suits to wear on other occasions. The environment of
a place is built up by the thought, feeling, etc. of the people who
congregate there. You will find a church has a particularly devotional
atmosphere taking on the atmosphere of the worshippers. A Lodge room
has an atmosphere peculiar to itself. Such places should never be
used for any other purpose. The custom of having religious services
in temples which are never entered for any other purpose, is most desirable. Likewise the Oriental custom of taking off the shoes and
going barefoot in the Temple is most proper, inasmuch as it helps to
remove the influence of the outer world. If the people do not go
barefoot in the Temple they should don slippers such as are used in
the Temple, and these should never be put on anywhere else. It may
even be found advisable to take a bath before beginning religious

service, in fact, where one can conveniently do so, it will be found advantageous.

Now, it may occur to the student to ask what all this has to do with Healing. It is simply to show that everything with which we come in contact becomes magnetized by our magnetism; that everything we touch is thus magnetized. It is for this reason that the American custom of handshaking is so very undesirable.

Now, inasmuch as everything we touch becomes magnetized by reason of our proximity to it and is capable of transmitting this magnetism to any one else who comes in contact with or proximity to it, logically it follows that articles may be deliberately magnetized for the express purpose of exercising this influence; that we may thus communicate healing virtues to an article so that it may be used in this way.

The Roman Catholic custom of blessing rosaries, crosses, crucifixes and other articles is, therefore, perfectly right and proper. The article will impart the influence that is given to it in the ceremony of blessing.

The custom of blessing houses, dedicating temples, churches, etc., is perfectly right and proper for it really and truly imparts an influence to them at the time of the blessing. The custom of blessing children is also perfectly right and proper, exercising this influence. But not only can we impart spiritual blessings, but may also impart physical blessings. We may impart a healing virtue to everything we bless. The habit of blessing food at the table is not an antiquated proceeding, not something that should be done away with as soon as possible, but is a custom having the greatest value, a custom that will exercise the greatest influence toward vitalizing the food, spiritualizing it and giving it a nutritive quality which does not naturally exist in it.

The therapeutic use of sacraments is one of the greatest agents in the healing art. A very good way is to take a napkin and hold it between the hands; then concentrate the mind in deep concentration; give a suggestive treatment to that napkin — just what it is to do, what influence it is to exercise, the effect it is to have, this treatment of blessing, should last five to ten minutes. In this way it becomes literally stirred up with the magnetic force, having the vibration to produce the effects thought into it at the time you are treating it. Then place the napkin on the patient at the place where the trouble is located, in pretty much the same manner you use a cloth saturated with liniment or a plaster or anything of that kind, or you may place it over the plexus controlling that part of the body. Let the patient wear it for awhile — fifteen minutes to half an hour; it will do no harm if he puts it on and wears it all night; in that way the treatment will go on all night. This will answer till the magnetism becomes exhausted. Then, of course, the patient will require a new napkin; that is one freshly magnetized.

You may magnetize a bandage and with it bandage a wound, and it will have a thousand times the healing effect that an ordinary bandage will have.

You may take a ring and bless it in the same way, holding it in your hand and concentrating on the effect it is to have, and then when it has been placed upon the hand of the patient, so soon as it is worn it will have the same influence. It should be borne in mind, also, that a ring may be magnetized so that it will transmit whatever influence is projected into it, whatever vibration you give to it will be transmitted to the body of the patient while wearing it.

You may take a garment and bless it in the same way and then have the patient wear it and it will transmit that healing force and heal the body of the patient. One of the greatest agents in this method is the use of magnetized water which may be magnetized in two or three different ways. One method is to take a rod and hold one end of it in the water, the other end in your hand and then transmit the force, give the blessing and allow the magnetism, the vibration to run into the water, down the rod, then have the patient drink of the water at different times; just as he would medicine and it will go through his entire body and exercise the healing force.

Again, you may place your hands over the water in a vessel and while holding the hands over it, give the blessing and transmit the healing magnetism through the air, having, of course, only a very small space between your fingers and the water, charging it in that way.

Again, you may place the water in a vessel and place your hands on the sides of the vessel, and while concentrating the mind, bless the water, imparting to it the healing efficacy. Likewise you may place a napkin over the water and by imparting the magnetism to the napkin, it may enter the water in this way.

Another method is simply to look at the water and while gazing at it, transmit the healing force.

Still another method is to breathe upon the water and while doing so transmit to it the magnetic power.

All these methods may be used and then the water given the same as an ordinary medicine, the water receiving its therapeutic value through the magical incantation said over it.

You may magnetize a piece of cloth by breathing on it as well as by placing the hands upon it. In that case, you should draw in your breath, fill your lungs full of air and then, as you breathe out, will for the cloth to receive certain healing powers and it will certainly receive them.

Relics, crucifixes, or anything of that kind may be blessed in such a way as to exercise a healing rather than a spiritualizing influence.

You may make use of this principle ad infinitum and it will exercise its influence to a high degree of perfection.

You may also magnetize a sheet of paper, of parchment. To do this you should place your hands on it and then make the affirmations and blessings. You may also blow your breath over it, imparting the blessing.

An object may be blessed by certain ceremonies as well as simply by a person placing his hands upon it. You may take a bit of parchment and bless it in this way or, in fact, by any of these methods, then take a new pen, which has never been used before, and a fresh bottle of ink, one that has not been opened before, so as to be sure there is no other magnetism there, or if you use an old pen, use one that has never been used for any purpose other than some kind of spiritual writing, and then write certain words or symbols on the parchment, such as cause to arouse in your mind the proper affirmations, such as will be in themselves an affirmation of what you want to take place, such as will compel you to affirm those things in the very act of thinking of them. By doing this you will impart to that a certain magnetic force, and a certain vibration.

The Jewish custom of wearing Phylacteries is really a survival of an understanding of this principle. The phylacteries are used for the purpose of transmitting the healing force. When a relic is used for healing purposes for a long time, the faith of the devotees imparts to it a healing virtue which all receive who come in contact with it and they in turn bless it.

The use of such articles is one of the greatest healing forces in nature. There is nothing that man can do, which is so valuable as the use of phylacteries, relics, etc.

It may occur to the student to ask why it would not be just as well to give a treatment. Well, in many instances it is not practical to do this. In many instances the patient lives at a vast distance or is in such condition that he cannot call upon the healer. The healer may find it difficult to reach the patient. Now, he can bless an article while he is giving a treatment, and that article will last quite a while and if worn, will continue to impart the healing virtue until that virtue has all passed to the body of the patient. The most of the healing virtue received in a treatment is thrown off. Frequently only a small percentage of it remains with the patient, but when an article is used, the treatment goes on for hours and days. However, it should be borne in mind that in sending articles by mail or express, to be used in this way, a great deal of care is necessary. The article should be wrapped in at least ten thicknesses of black silk, thoroughly wrapped so that there is no possibility of the magnetism escaping, silk acting as a non-conductor. It should then be put in a package, carefully sealed and sent. It will be better, however, if it can be committed to the hands of a person, one of faith and spirituality. Much care, however, must be exercised in transmitting these articles to see that their healing virtue is not sapped by the one who handles them; likewise that his magnetism is not imparted to them.

If people would learn to have their clothes ceremonially blessed before putting them on, to have every article which they bring into their homes blessed, having everything they come in contact with, be thoroughly magnetized, they would find it would lead to their spiritual, mental, emotional and physical health in a much greater degree than they have any idea.

This principle may be resorted to in a systematic manner as a means of relieving practically every disease to which flesh is heir. As a matter of fact, Magnetic Healing, Psychical, Spiritual and Divine Healing may all be imparted through those magnetized objects.

Also, the same method as used by the high potency homeopath may be used in this way. All the power of suggestion may also be transmitted. Haven't you ever realized that as soon as you touch certain objects, whether you know anything about their past history, or not, thoughts which have been foreign to you, come to you. Sometimes they are good and sometimes bad. Well, it is because of the magnetism existing within the article. Objects may be used as a means of suggestion. Whenever they are looked upon or approached they will transmit this suggestive influence to the consciousness of the patient, and it may in this way be employed as a means of transmitting therapeutic influences to the organism of the patient.

Magical Therapeutics is, therefore, not imagination, not guess work, but is an exact science, based upon the fundamental principles of Magnetism, based upon the great truth that everything we touch is magnetized whether or not we will it, that, therefore, when our minds are concentrated we shall be able to transmit the healing current with a hundredfold greater strength than would ordinarily take place, and this current being imparted to the organism of every one who comes in contact with it, may thus be utilized as a means of healing.

The Rituals of all religions and of all fraternities, etc., admit this principle. It was employed by the early Christians, and is employed today by many healers and spiritualists. For this reason it is of great importance that it should be made use of systematically and intelligently by those who understand the reason why it exercises these influences.

The foregoing will give the student a perfectly accurate comprehension of the principle involved, a realization of the laws underlying

the operations of magnetism through these objects. As a result he will
be able to systematically employ it in the healing of disease.

L E S S O N
O N
P S Y C H I C   D I A G N O S I S

It is of the greatest importance to the Healer to always be able to diagnose the case of a patient. If he does not know the nature of the trouble he will not be in a proper position to treat the patient.

Physical diagnosis is not always satisfactory owing to the fact that the trouble which must be dealt with is very often more deep seated than the physical being, as we have seen. It may be a disorder of the Mental Body, the Astral Body, the Vital Force or Etheric Double and quite often an improper condition in the soul and physical diagnosis, of course, will never manifest a trouble of this kind. We must look deeper in order to find the source of the trouble, and in order to apply Metaphysical Methods of Healing, it is necessary to know the cause back of the physical manifestation, therefore, a Metaphysical method of diagnosis is necessary to the ascertaining of the Metaphysical source of the trouble, in order that we may apply metaphysical methods of treatment.

Another difficulty in ordinary diagnosis is the fact that the cause of disease given in the medical books are of little value in metaphysical treatment. We do not regard disease as an entity or as an original trouble. Disease is really an effort on the part of Nature to purge out a poison accumulated in the system and in its very nature it is also a manifestation of a disturbance. He must get at the root of the matter in order to know just how to go about the treatment and in order to get at the root of the matter we must have some purely psychical method of diagnosis. We must know just what the trouble is, and we fortunately have a method of psychical diagnosis that perfectly informs us of the trouble, with the cause of the disease so that we may be enabled to apply proper methods of treatment.

Inasmuch as the cause of all states of health and disease is specifically a state of vibration, harmonious if it produces health, discordant if producing disease, it follows that in order to ascertain the ultimate cause of the symptoms, we must know just what that state of vibration is. In Psychometry we have a perfect method. The Psychometric sensitive really takes on the condition of the patient for the time being and by taking on the patient's condition, the very vibration that is operative in the patient's aura is brought into his own. He senses the patient's condition for the simple reason that he is subject to that condition himself for the time being. For the time being, he has the disease, therefore, he feels just as the patient feels. He is not diagnosing objectively, but subjectively. In this way he is able to feel just where the trouble is in the patient. He does not treat names of diseases, but he does treat the pathological condition which is the effect of a disturbed vibratory state, and he knows what this disturbed vibratory state is because he feels it. He is in the same position as the patient, therefore, he is able, by a process of self diagnosis, to ascertain with perfect accuracy, the trouble. Knowing now, where the patient suffers, knowing what his condition is, he knows intellectually just what the trouble is with the patient, and is able to go to work and relieve it. However, this method is very dangerous for the reason that you actually have those vibrations operating in your system, you have the cause, the very germ of the patient's trouble, established in your own Aura, and if you are not careful to throw it off as soon as the diagnosis is completed, if you allow this disturbed vibration to remain with you, it is only a question of time before it will develop the corresponding disease. It is in this way that many healing mediums also many Christian Scientists have contracted the diseases of their patients at the same time curing the patients. The patient gets well; the disease passes to the healer because in diagnosis he has taken on the condition of the patient, and failed to throw it off. The proper method for psychical diagnosis is to remain perfectly negative, drawing on to yourself the condition of the patient, drawing his Aura into your own and remain two or three minutes in this condition — five minutes will not harm seriously, and then, having realized the trouble, knowing what you want to know, become intensely positive, cause a wave to pass outward from the center of your being, with an outward projection of the will, so that the condition is entirely thrown off and your Aura is cleaned from it. In this way you will be able to protect yourself, to purge yourself of the influence and will be safe.

It is not always necessary, however, to take on the condition. By sensing it you may be able to know what the condition is, by responding to the vibration, without altogether taking on the condition. Of course, this will not be quite so reliable as taking on the patient's condition. A very good way to diagnose psychometrically is to take the patient by the hand, even by both hands and by concentrating negatively for a few seconds, cease all thought and try to feel what comes to you. When you give way to this feeling that comes upon you, receiving whatever impressions you get at this time, it must be relied upon. If you take on the condition you will feel in that part of your body the trouble, otherwise, you will only get an impression of what the trouble may be.

A good way to diagnose psychometrically is to go through the good old dodge of feeling the patient's pulse, examining his tongue, etc., take hold of the patient by the wrist with the fingers; then, becoming negative as possible, count his pulse beat and after you have put in about as much time as you can safely at that, still holding his hand, ask to see his tongue and then ask about how regularly his bowels move and all those hackneyed questions about diagnosis, but really pay no attention to the answers which he gives. You may take his temperature while you are going through the "Rig-ama-role" — but sense the vibration, note the impressions that come to you. You may take on his condition or you may simply get certain ideas, but the ideas that occur to you, or impressions, must be relied on absolutely. There is nothing quite so reliable as the impressions received in this psychical diagnosis.

Another very good way to diagnose is to use an article, the same as in psychometric reading. Take a handkerchief or a ring that the patient has carried, or worn, a collar, a necktie, if it be a gentleman, or a lady's fan, a piece of jewelry — anything of the kind, a lock of hair, anything that the patient has handled a great deal and something which others have not handled. Simply hold the article in the hand as you would in giving a psychometric reading, and note the impressions that come to you. You may either take on the condition of the person or else simply give expression to the thoughts that come to you. In either case, however, you proceed exactly as in giving a psychometric reading, in fact, it is a psychometric reading you are giving. You pay no attention to the impressions you receive of a spiritual character, nothing of that kind or the ordinary fortune-telling impressions. You simply note those relating to the patient's state of health; then you know what the trouble is and can act accordingly.

One great advantage of this style of diagnosis is the fact that you can diagnose without the patient's knowing anything about it. His friends may come to you and bring an article and you may psychometrize it and thus know his condition. Then when he comes to you, instead of asking him any questions or psychometrizing an article, or anything, you can simply tell him what is the matter with him and there is nothing in the world that so inspires confidence in the healer on the part of the patient, as the ability to look into the heart of the patient and tell him what the trouble is, and there is nothing so important as the credulity of the patient, in fact you may employ this

psychometric dodge without the agency of his relatives. When a gentleman comes into your office, politely ask him to let you have his hat
and in a very polite manner, hang it up on a rack, do not allow him to
do it himself, and while you are hanging it up, be intensely negative
and catch the vibrations. When you have had sufficient practice, you
can diagnose his case while you are hanging his hat up. Then tell him
specifically what the matter is, tell him you do not want him to say a
word, but tell him his trouble, and do not spare him, tell him all
about it. If it be a case of syphilis tell him he has it and if he deny
it, tell him he is a liar and not to try to fool you, give him distinctly to understand that you know just what you are talking about,
that you see into his life; he concludes then that he has found his
prophet, and it is very important as a means of suggestion. Nothing
establishes confidence in your ability to cure disease like the ability
to know WHAT IT IS.

Again if one of your lady patients comes into your office, in-
sist upon hanging up her cloak for her, or something of the kind, or
use some bit of gallantry, if nothing more than giving her a glass of
wine, or a glass of water, or something of the kind, anything to come
in contact with her in some way, and the moment you do, drink in the condition and then you know how to proceed.

Not only, however, is it possible to diagnose in this way, but
with practice, you can get so you can diagnose while shaking hands
with a person. When a person comes in, rise and in a very polite manner, give the good hearty, free and easy American handshake and while
doing it, be negative, but draw on his magnetism whatever you do. If a
child comes in, it is advisable to lay your hands on his head in a real
fatherly way and ask how he is feeling, etc., and while you are doing
this, diagnose his case and then deal with the case accordingly.

Also, by becoming negative the moment a patient comes into your
office, it is possible to diagnose a case without touching the patient,
even when entirely across the room. You can draw the Aura into you,
respond to it until you feel the vibration and in this way you can
sense the condition being enabled to tell just what the trouble is
and then you can act accordingly. Whatever impression you get while
in this negative state, should be relied upon, only you may possibly
catch the thought he has, if it come in the form of an intellectual
impression, but this will not be the case if you take on the condition
so as to feel the trouble, as he feels it.

Psychometry is always more reliable than any other form of diagnosis because you can feel as the patient feels. However, it is not
the only form of psychical diagnosis. By developing Clairolfacious-
ness, you can diagnose the patient's trouble by means of the odor
emanating from him. You can smell out his disease, in other words.
Bear in mind that each disease has a particular odor peculiar to itself.

Owing to the fact that all disease is a manifestation of a certain form of discordant vibration always manifesting in odor as well as in form, color, sound, etc., you are able by developing this sense sufficiently, to smell the different odors and with practice, you can associate those different odors with different diseases. This, however, cannot be followed intuitively. It requires practice. You must know what the odors will be. Generally speaking very offensive odors, everything in the form of a stench, is a manifestation of disease, while the perfumes represent health and the finer perfumes much more than a normal state of health. Take, for instance, venereal diseases. There is nothing in the world so abominably stinking as the odor emanating from the Aura of a person who has abused the sex organs and has contracted venereal disease and particularly the form manifested as syphilis, gonorrhoea, etc. The syphilitic odor is a kind of sour stench. On the other hand, one who has not abused the sex principle, a virgin, in fact, who has a well developed sexual organism, and no disease bothering in any way, but who is strongly sexed, emanates the most wonderful perfume conceiveable. As a matter of fact, the use of perfume by women is invariably resorted to as a means of counteracting the odor from the sexual Aura. The woman whose sexual system is in proper shape, will never resort to perfumes. She does not have to. These odors are very often sensed by the physical sense of smell, though the finer odors, those finer differentiations, can be sensed only through the psychical senses. In time, however, you will be able to classify the diverse states by means of sensing the odors emanating from them.

Again, by developing Clairgustience, you can diagnose psychically, through the taste. This is particularly valuable in ascertaining the chemical condition of the being and discovering the Astral, Etheric and Mental Chemistry of the system. When you are diagnosing a case psychically and there comes into your mouth a taste exactly corresponding to the taste of crude chemical, a taste which reminds you of that chemical, be sure you are sensing the presence of that chemical in the system of some of the higher principles.

Thus, by tasting of the Aura, you are able to tell of the Chemicals that are in the system. While diagnosing a case if your teeth become gritty, just as if taking iron, know that there is a superabundance of iron in the system and if you have a bitter taste in the mouth, know that some bitter chemical is present. You have to develop this power until you can distinguish the different bitterness and whatever it may be. You can recognize too much sugar, trace sugar poisoning in the system by an extremely sweet taste. You can recognize too much acid when you have a very tart taste, particularly if sufficient to set your teeth on edge. In time, you will be able to diagnose almost any condition in this way, but you do not have to depend on these methods either, for you will develop Clairvoyance, by practice, so that you can look into the Aura of your patient and see the colors present in the Aura. You can thus diagnose the disease of your patient providing you know how to interpret those colors. The colors, of course, symbolize different states of health and you must be able to diagnose the states by interpreting the meaning of those colors; likewise, you can develop the power to see the figures that appear in the Aura as it vibrates; the forms that play back and forth in it and in this way you will be enabled to ascertain the vibration. Of course, to do this you must have a knowledge of the forms that will appear. In regard to color diagnosis, it may be briefly stated that dull colors indicate a slugglish condition of the system – the activity is low, there is a sinking, as it were, a lack of activity; while a bright color indicates extreme activity. Again, rose being the color of Prana, the presence of rose color in the Aura will, of course indicate vital force while total absence of the rose color will indicate a very low state of vitality. Again, pink will indicate a good physical condition, while physical degeneracy will be indicated by absence of the pink color. Likewise, it may be stated that lead poison will make the color of the Aura very dark, approaching black, and in fact, the different metals will give their corresponding colors. Iron will make a color approaching very nearly a ruby tint, a red approaching the color of the ruby.

Mercury will produce usually a green cast as it comes in the Aura because it is not a physical mercury that we are now dealing with, that is not what manifests, but the higher forms; it will be very often green perhaps, in certain conditions approaching yellow. A negative condition of the Aura, that is a magnetic condition, will be indicated by the absence of red, and the presence of blue, if it be in the Astral Body, and in the Etheric Double also by a pale color or approaching green, and where the life force instead of having the bright color, has a color approaching green. White will also indicate a magnetic state while red or gold will indicate the electrical condition in a general sense.

By making use of these methods of diagnosis you will be able to ascertain the condition of your patient in reference to vibration. Having realized his vibratory state you can then proceed to restore the condition of his system to what it should be. It should here be recognized, however, that we are not treating names of diseases. We are treating states of vibration. In order, therefore, to apply psychical diagnosis properly to the healing of diseases we must know the vibratory state and know how to correct it, and by resorting to this psychical method we will be enabled to ascertain that vibratory state and in time, to apply the proper remedy and bring about the desired state of harmony.

As disease is discord and health is harmony, disease can be cured only by replacing discord with harmony. Likewise we must know the particular phase of discord in order to restore harmony. In order to know this, we must be able to sense it. We can not approach it by any signs or evidences through any system of physical diagnosis, but must sense that particular vibration by psychical diagnosis. In this way we can proceed with absolute accuracy. Psychical Diagnosis is well nigh infallible, while physical diagnosis is far from such.

CPSIA information can be obtained
at www.ICGtesting.com
Printed in the USA
BVHW010602051220
594911BV00010B/71